PALEO FOR BEGINNERS

Rockridge Press

CONTENTS

Chapter 4: A Week of Preparation—Ready, Set, Go!

Chapter 5: 7-Day Meal Plan 45

Chapter 6: Breakfasts

Chapter 7: Soups, Salads, and Dressings

Chapter 8: Main Dishes

Chapter 9: Side Dishes and Sauces

Chapter 10: Desserts and Snacks

Conclusion 189

Index 190

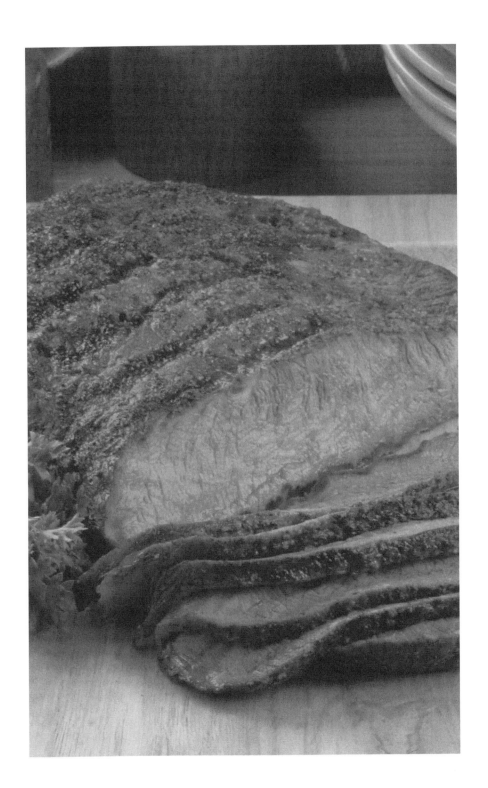

1

WHAT IS THE PALEO DIET?

The Paleo diet has become incredibly popular in the past few years, leading many people to assume that it's a new way of eating. In reality, the Paleo diet has been around for almost forty years.

How the Paleo Diet Came About

In 1975, a gastroenterologist named Dr. Walter Voegtlin published a book called *The Stone Age Diet*. In the book, he documented how he treated patients with a diet that replicated the eating patterns of people during the Paleolithic era. The diet prescribed consuming large quantities of animal fats and proteins and very small quantities of carbohydrates. Dr. Voegtlin reported that his patients, who suffered from disorders such as Crohn's disease and irritable bowel syndrome, showed significant health improvements when following the diet.

Unfortunately, *The Stone Age Diet* didn't make much headway with the public. At that time, almost everyone believed that a low-fat, low-calorie diet was the only healthy way to eat.

An Ancient Diet for Modern Times

Ten years later, however, Dr. S. Boyd Eaton and Dr. Melvin Konner published a paper in *The New England Journal of Medicine* that supported Dr. Voegtlin's research and that received a lot of attention from the medical community and the media. The popularity of their paper on the Paleolithic era diet led to the publication of their book, *The Paleolithic Prescription: A Program of Diet & Exercise and a Design for Living*. This book established the principles most variations of the Paleo diet follow today.

The book explained the way our Paleolithic ancestors ate and why that nutritional lifestyle was such a healthy one. The most important thing the authors accomplished was to make the ancient diet suitable for modern times. The book laid out the nutritional content of the original Paleolithic diet and then showed readers how to get that nutritional profile from modern and widely available foods. It was an adaptable way to eat like our ancestors, and it paved the way for today's Paleo diet phenomenon.

The Paleo Diet for You, the Modern Cave-Dweller

There are several versions of the Paleo diet around today; these versions generally differ in terms of how strictly they follow the eating patterns of our Paleolithic ancestors. The Paleo diet described in this book is a version that intends to closely duplicate the nutritional makeup of a Paleolithic diet without being unrealistic, difficult or complicated. You'll reap the health and weight loss benefits of the Paleo diet without having to turn your entire lifestyle inside out or spend time searching for exotic ingredients. You'll be practicing a diet that is moderate in its approach, but you will likely see incredible results.

What the Paleo Diet Looks Like

The Paleo diet is designed to duplicate the results and benefits of our pre-agricultural diet without duplicating the diet's prehistoric methods. While there are a few Paleo followers who do literally hunt, gather or forage all of their food, most people don't have the motivation or time for that level of authenticity. Fortunately, we can achieve the same Paleolithic results with foods readily available to us in grocery stores, health foods stores and farmers markets.

The Paleo diet food pyramid is an inverted version of the one that used to be recommended by the USDA. Meats, eggs and seafood make up the majority of the day's calories, followed by fats from plant foods, fruits and vegetables, and then nuts and seeds. The Paleo diet is a high-protein/low-carbohydrate diet.

Chapter 2 will go into more detail on what you'll be eating from each food group and also give you a specific list of allowed (and disallowed) foods. For now, we'll cover the basics.

What Is Not on Your Paleo Plate?

The Paleo diet is effective not only because of what you eat, but also because of what you don't eat. Changing the components and proportions of your diet is only half the Paleo plan. The other half involves eliminating foods that can slow your metabolism, encourage blood sugar problems and fat storage, and slow digestion. These eliminated foods include processed foods, alcohol, grains, legumes and sugar.

Processed Foods

Fast food, frozen meals and store-bought sweets and snacks are not a part of the Paleo diet and should be avoided.

Alcohol

Not only was alcohol an unlikely component of a Paleolithic-era diet, but it is also filled with empty calories and sugar. Alcohol does not supply enough nutritional value to offset its negative dietary attributes, and therefore is not included in the Paleo diet.

Grains

Grains, including all breads, pasta, rice, oats and barley, are agricultural products; you are embarking on a pre-agricultural diet. Later this chapter will explain in greater detail why grains are specifically off-limits.

Legumes

As with grains, legumes such as beans, peas, soy and soy derivatives are agricultural products and are therefore off-limits. The specific risks to your health that these foods pose will be explained later in this chapter.

Sugar

One of the remarkable things about the Paleo diet is the impact it can have not only on lowering blood sugar levels, but also on decreasing your risk of developing diabetes and metabolic syndrome. In part, this is because sugars are eliminated on the Paleo diet. It is also very important to avoid substituting artificial sweeteners for sugar. You can, however, use honey in moderation, as it was likely a part of the ancestral diet.

What Is on Your Paleo Plate?

Meats, Eggs and Seafood

This food group is where you will get most of your calories. All meat, fish, shellfish, mollusks and eggs are allowed, but there are some guidelines for choosing the right foods for the best results. The most important thing is that these foods are of high quality and are prepared with Paleo-approved ingredients.

Fats from Plant Sources

These sources include olives and olive oil, avocadoes (which are a fruit but serve as a fat), and nuts and seeds (which are described in detail in the next section). Since butter is a dairy product and does not improve your heart health, it should be avoided when cooking or preparing foods; use pure olive oil for cooking and grape-seed oil or extra virgin olive oil for uncooked dressings.

Nuts and Seeds

Nuts and seeds were a big part of the Paleolithic-era diet. All nuts are allowed, with the exception of peanuts, which are a legume. Seeds are allowed, including flax seeds, sunflower seeds, pumpkin seeds, sesame seeds and others. If you are frightened by the idea of giving up pasta and rice, the good news is that quinoa is allowed. Not only is quinoa a seed, but it also makes a great substitute for rice, pasta, oats, barley and other grain foods.

Fruits and Vegetables

The fruits allowed on the Paleo diet are those that would have been readily available (foraged) in the pre-agricultural era. These foraged fruits include berries, such as cranberries, raspberries, strawberries and blueberries. Tree fruits are also a mainstay of the Paleo diet; they include citrus fruits, apples, peaches, plums, cherries, nectarines and pears.

Condiments

Some condiments are allowed, but they should be limited to those that do not contain sugar or any of the forbidden ingredients. Ketchup, for example, is not allowed; mustard, on the other hand, is made from seeds and usually does not contain added sugar. In general, try to rely on herbs and spices rather than condiments.

Beverages

Allowed beverages include pure fruit and vegetable juices, but they should be unsweetened versions and consumed in moderation. Water should be your primary beverage. Tea and coffee are acceptable on the Paleo diet, as long as you use almond milk to lighten them, rather than dairy milk.

Losing Weight on the Paleo Diet

For years, many mainstream dieticians and healthcare providers have touted the benefits of cutting out most meats and oils (because of their fat content) and eliminating some fruits and vegetables (because of their natural carbohydrate content). They've also strongly advocated eating large quantities of grains and legumes (for their high fiber content).

These nutritionists have insisted that a diet low in calories and fat is the only way to maintain good health and lose weight. However, the research behind the Paleo diet indicates that this isn't the case. Paleolithic diet research shows that a diet rich in healthy fats and proteins and low in sugars and starches is not only extremely healthy, but also an excellent way to lose weight.

How Does It Work?

You may be wondering: How can I lose weight when I'm still eating meats, fats and high-carb fruits and veggies?

The answer: By using the Paleo methods to align your diet with your body's historical genetic programming, you can boost your metabolic rate, speed healthy and complete digestion, regulate some of the hormones related to energy and fat storage, and reduce hunger and cravings for unhealthy foods.

The foods you'll be eating on the Paleo diet are the ones our bodies have been programmed to eat for tens of thousands of years. The foods you're eliminating from your diet are foods we've only been eating for the last one percent of recorded human history; foods that, according to the Paleo diet, are ones that we are not (yet) genetically adapted to eat. These "new" foods slow digestion and metabolism, wreak havoc with our hormones, and cause our bodies to both overeat and store excess fat.

If history serves as a guide, your body needs the good fats, vitamins, minerals, fiber and carbs it gets from meats, fruits, vegetables, nuts and seeds. But it does not need modern grains, legumes or sugars. If you examine the health of the few cultures that still follow this type of diet, you'll see that they are healthier, leaner and tend to live longer than those of us who eat diets heavy in sugar, grains and processed foods.

Why Many Low-Fat, High-Carb Diets Fail

If you're trying to lose weight, the chances are good that this isn't the first time you've tried to do so. Many of us do our best to find the perfect diet and follow it to a T. We may even successfully lose weight for a short time, but do so at the cost of personal comfort— and often at the cost of good health. When you deprive yourself of adequate protein and fats, you're likely to be hungry.

Another problem with mainstream diets is that the grains they recommend are high in starches, which our bodies quickly convert to sugar. The rapid starch-to-sugar conversion process is a common cause of blood sugar spikes, which are quickly followed by blood sugar crashes. These crashes can cause fatigue, lethargy and a craving for more starchy carbs to help pick us back up.

The main problem with these mainstream diets is that many people fail to stick with them for long periods of time. A common reason for this failure is carb-driven cravings. Eliminating carbs, and therefore these cravings, is one of the biggest benefits of the Paleo diet.

Why the Paleo Diet Works

There are a few major differences between how the Paleo diet works and how other diets work. These differences are important because they are likely to directly affect your odds of success in losing weight.

- Low-glycemic carbs that you eat from plant sources can help reduce cravings and increase your energy level.

- High-fiber foods can help keep you full longer, especially if they don't contain the starches that are present in grains.

- Protein contributes to building lean muscle, which can help you burn fat faster.

- Omega-3 fatty acids and other healthy fats can help make you feel full, slow your body's metabolism of sugars, keep your blood sugar levels steady, and help you burn stored fat.

- Increased vitamin C from fresh fruits and vegetables, especially berries, can help your body metabolize fat. The process of metabolizing fat results in burning existing stored fat as fuel and using the fat you eat for energy instead of storing it.

- A low-sugar diet can help you avoid insulin resistance and blood sugar level fluctuations. Steadier blood sugar levels can help keep your energy level constant and reduce fatigue.

As these points show, a major benefit of the Paleo diet is that you'll be unlikely to feel deprived of food or energy. Since the Paleo diet doesn't involve calorie counting, you won't find yourself worrying about a tablespoon of this or one-third of a cup of that. Instead, your primary concern will be to avoid the modern foods that your body can't digest efficiently.

Why You Need Fat to Lose Fat

Why would you need to eat more fats to lose weight? It's a common question. And the idea that you should eat more dietary fat to lose body fat certainly does sound odd. But it's the *type* of fat you're eating that leads to weight loss (or gain). One type of fat that drives weight loss are the omega-3 fatty acids. These fatty acids are often referred to as "essential" because your body needs them to function properly but is unable to produce them on its own. To get your required amounts of omega-3 fatty acids, you need to either get them from the foods you eat or take a supplement.

One of the main ways omega-3s affect body weight is by regulating insulin production. A common cause of a "belly" or fatty midsection is an insulin-related inability to properly metabolize sugar into glucose, which then fails to be properly converted into glycogen. When the body fails to convert glucose into glycogen, which would then be converted into energy, it stores the excess glucose as fat.

The role of omega-3 fatty acids in this process is to enable the body to produce the chemicals that are necessary to ultimately convert glucose into energy. If you're not getting enough of these essential fatty acids, it becomes more difficult for your body to perform this conversion task optimally. On the Paleo diet, you'll be eating foods laden with omega-3 fatty acids, such as grass-fed meats, seafood, nuts and seeds. While you can get these fatty acids from supplements, incorporating them into your diet naturally is ideal.

All Proteins Are Not the Same

The difference between consuming the processed hamburgers and hot dogs that are forbidden on the Paleo diet and the lean steaks and salmon that are recommended could be the difference between obesity and a leaner, healthier you. There are three main attributes of meats that can affect not only the speed with which you will lose weight, but also your odds of keeping the weight off in the long term.

- **The type and quality of the fats.** Cheap hamburgers and processed meats such as hot dogs often have added low-quality saturated fats to boost their weight and flavor. While lean steaks and salmon may contain the same amount of fats, they are good fats—the omega-3 fatty acids and other healthy fats your body needs to function properly.

- **The quality and digestibility of the proteins.** Low-end and processed meats usually contain lower amounts of protein and it is of poor quality. High-quality meats and fish contain high amounts of lean protein that your body can easily extract, digest and use to build muscle.

- **The addition of fillers and preservatives.** Processed meats are typically full of fillers and preservatives that add calories, adversely affect your health, and contribute to weight gain. Lean proteins such as filet mignon don't contain these additives and preservatives.

By changing the quality of the proteins that you eat, you're likely to notice a difference in how you look and feel. You may also lose weight and find that your muscles gain additional tone and definition. You'll probably feel fuller, longer when you eat high-quality protein, as it takes your body longer to digest it. These incentives are some of the many for eating the best proteins available.

Summary: Losing Weight on the Paleo Diet

The Paleo diet has several key advantages for people who are looking for a safe, effective way to lose weight and keep it off. The diet recommends consuming lean proteins and fats that help build lean muscle and convert sugars into glycogen that your body can use as energy. It also recommends eliminating sugar, alcohol and processed foods that can make you sick and overweight.

The Paleo diet isn't meant to be a short-term weight loss method. It's a change in lifestyle that many—particularly those previously eating a modern diet—find leads to long-term weight loss.

Better Health Through the Paleo Diet

While used by many people today as a way to lose weight, the Paleo diet was originally intended to realign humans with their natural, historical way of eating. As a result of this realignment, the diet's goals were to restore good health and avoid the modern diseases that are potentially tied to modern diets.

What's the Theory Behind the Paleo Diet?

The Paleo diet's original creator, Dr. Walter L. Voegtlin, believed humans aren't genetically designed to digest the modern grains, dairy products, sugars and all of the processed food that we exist on today. Instead, he believed our bodies operate best when running on foods such as lean meats, fish, shellfish, eggs, nuts, veggies, fruits and honey—the only foods we consumed and relied on until the Neolithic agricultural revolution approximately 10,000 years ago. Dr. Voegtlin's theory was subsequently supported by the results he saw in his patients and by decades of respected research that followed.

It's only in the past several thousand years, and in some cases only the past several decades, that we've added sugars, alcohol, grains, and engineered and/or processed foods to our diets. As a result, we're suffering from modern diseases commonly referred to as "diseases of affluence" at increasing rates. These diseases are likely the result of our bodies' inability to digest these modern foods.

Preventing or Reversing Metabolic Syndrome

Metabolic syndrome is a group of risk factors that increase the odds of developing diseases such as type 2 diabetes, stroke and heart disease. Risk factors include:

- Extra weight around the waist (for men, a waist of 40 inches or more; for women, 35 inches or more)

- Low HDL cholesterol (for men, under 40 mg/dL; for women, under 50 mg/dL)

- High blood pressure (higher than 130/85 mm Hg)

- High triglycerides (higher than 150 mg/dL)

- High fasting blood sugar (higher than 100 mg/DL)

If three or more of these risk factors are present, you are considered to have metabolic syndrome.

The Paleo diet helps reduce and/or prevent the incidence of these factors by eliminating the foods shown to contribute to these illnesses, including refined sugar, white flour and processed, fatty foods. Combined with increased consumption of lean proteins and healthy fats, a decrease in metabolic syndrome risk is likely.

Improved Heart Health

Improved heart health is one of the biggest reasons the Paleo diet has garnered so much attention from the medical community. The lean proteins and good fats of the Paleo diet are essential for heart health.

Because the Paleo diet recommends lean meats, shellfish and fish that are low in the unhealthy saturated fats, it can help lower bad cholesterol and triglycerides and reduce or potentially reverse arteriosclerosis. Arteriosclerosis is one of the leading causes of stroke, blood clots and aneurysms.

Improved Digestive Health

Because the Paleo diet eliminates most processed grains and legumes, diseases such as colitis, celiac disease, irritable bowel syndrome and Crohn's disease are less likely to develop, and those with these illnesses may find their symptoms reduced. The diet encourages you to consume fibrous foods such as fruits and vegetables that help flush your digestive system and keep your colon clean and clear. Digestive issues such as diarrhea, constipation, chronic gas, heartburn, acid reflux and GERD (gastroesophageal reflux disease) are often reduced or eliminated after following the diet for a sustained time period.

Maximized Immune System

Eliminating foods that our bodies aren't genetically equipped to digest will often reduce the incidence of allergies and other immune system issues. You may be surprised to learn that conditions such as lupus, fibromyalgia and rheumatoid arthritis are also considered to be disorders of the immune system. Some patients with these diseases who switched to the Paleo diet have reported positive results.

The Paleo diet is naturally gluten- and lactose-free; both are substances that some people's bodies treat as allergens. It also eliminates foods that contain other possible allergens, such as antibiotics, preservatives, hormones and dyes. This leaves your immune system increasingly available to fight off disease instead of constantly battling issues caused by foods.

Many people who begin the Paleo diet aren't aware that they're suffering from allergic symptoms until they notice the symptoms have disappeared. Some of these symptoms include frequent headaches, stuffy nose, nausea, swelling of the hands and feet, or general bloating and puffiness. All of these are common immune responses and may go away when you stop exposing your body to the wheat, flours, additives and other ingredients that could be causing them.

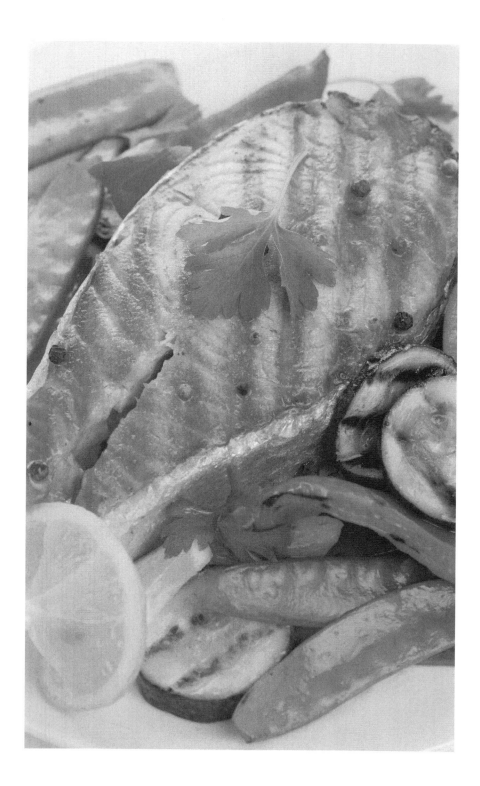

2

STARTING YOUR PALEO DIET

In this chapter we'll cover the foods of the Paleo diet in detail, including how and where to shop for them. This chapter will also show you how to plan Paleo meals day by day, so that you understand what you'll be eating. Finally, it will discuss some tips to help make your transition to the Paleo diet a smooth, enjoyable and successful one.

What You'll Be Eating on the Paleo Diet

Much of the success of the Paleo diet lies not only in the types of foods you eat, but also the quality of those foods. Our ancestors ate wild foods that were of high quality and free of chemicals, hormones and many other ingredients that have made the modern diet largely unhealthy.

For most people, the idea of raising, hunting and/or foraging for their own food is unrealistic. Many people also lack the budget for unusual (and therefore often expensive) ingredients. Taking these considerations into account, the following guidelines recommend Paleo-approved foods that are realistic to find and purchase.

Later this chapter will explain how to find these foods in your local supermarket and through other local resources.

Animal and Fish Proteins

Animal and fish proteins make up the majority of the Paleo diet. It is recommended that you purchase the highest quality proteins that you can reasonably afford. If wild game, exotic meats like buffalo, and wild salmon are too expensive for your budget, rest assured that grass-fed beef, organic chicken and fresh or frozen shrimp are just as good.

The Paleo diet recommends that livestock meats such as beef, buffalo, ostrich, pork and lamb are grass fed, organic, and free of any hormones or antibiotics. You are also encouraged to eat wild meat and game, such as deer and boar. When considering which cuts of meat to buy, lean cuts are preferred to cuts with a high fat content.

Poultry should be organic, vegetarian-raised and free of hormones. Chicken, turkey, duck, goose and Cornish hens are good Paleo options. Eggs are also an easy and excellent source of protein on the Paleo diet, but they should be from free-range, organic birds.

Your seafood choices are numerous. You can eat all kinds of fish, shrimp, crab, clams, oysters, lobster and other crustaceans and mollusks. It is recommended that you prioritize cold-water fish varieties such as cod, haddock, mackerel and salmon to maximize your omega-3 consumption.

You can prepare your meat, poultry and seafood by steaming, broiling, grilling, sautéing, pan-frying, baking or broiling. Avoid deep frying, because neither the batters nor the typical deep frying oils are recommended.

Fruits and Vegetables

There are a large number of delicious fruits and vegetables to choose from. In general, you can eat any fruits and vegetables other than corn and some root vegetables, which have a high sugar and starch content. Carrots can be eaten in moderation, and onions are historically a wild crop and therefore acceptable.

Try to select low-glycemic fruits and vegetables for most of your meals and snacks. In doing so, you'll be more likely to maintain an even blood sugar level and have a steadier source of energy.

Whenever possible, the fruits and vegetables you purchase (as well as mushrooms and other plant foods) should be organic and in season. This ensures that they are as healthy, nutritious and delicious as possible. Frozen fruits and vegetables are allowed, but you should keep them to a minimum. Canned fruits and vegetables are typically overcooked and over-salted, and should be avoided.

Nuts, Seeds and Oils

Nuts, seeds and oils are an important part of the Paleo diet. They supply healthy fats, fiber and a feeling of fullness that can help keep you from being besieged by unhealthy cravings.

Allowed nuts include tree nuts, such as pecans, walnuts and almonds. Peanuts are a legume and are therefore not allowed. Nuts should be eaten raw as often as possible; if you prefer roasted nuts, make sure they're roasted without sugar, salt or added oil. Seeds such as pumpkin seeds, sunflower seeds, squash seeds and sesame seeds make great snacks, and flax seed or flax seed oil is loaded with healthy fats and antioxidants.

Use extra virgin olive oil for making dressings, as a substitute for butter on veggies, and for cooking foods at low heat. Use pure olive oil or grape-seed oil for cooking at medium to high temperatures.

Shopping for Food on the Paleo Diet

You should be able to get the majority of your Paleo groceries from a good supermarket, particularly if you shop at a supermarket that has an extensive organics section.

The most important thing you can do to be successful shopping at a regular supermarket is to shop from the outer sections and skip the center aisles. Most grocery stores are set up with the meat, seafood and produce aisles on the perimeter of the store, while packaged and processed foods are often found in the center.

The following overview of supermarket departments will give you some ideas for how to shop Paleo at your local grocery store.

The Produce Department

A large portion of your groceries will come from this department. You want to shop seasonally as much as possible, as seasonal produce is at its peak of freshness and nutritional value. Local fruits and vegetables are often of better quality than those shipped from far away. Buy organic as much as possible. If your budget is tight and you need to be selective about your organic produce, the produce that you peel can be safely eaten non-organic.

Fruits and veggies that are darker in color—such as reds, oranges and yellows—are typically the highest in antioxidants and phytonutrients. Try to get as much produce in these darker colors as possible. It is also recommended to select dark green vegetables, particularly kale, spinach, broccoli, collards and other greens. Iceberg lettuce, on the other hand, is low in nutrients—opt for leaf lettuces or Romaine for your salads.

The Meat Department

Most supermarkets have an organic meat section, which is where you are recommended to do most of your meat shopping. There may also be some organic meats and seafood in the frozen foods section.

Read all packaging carefully to make sure your meat selections are organic and grass fed. Choose leaner cuts such as loins, leaner steaks and some roasts. You can occasionally eat fattier cuts, but keep your consumption to a minimum.

The Seafood Department

Try to buy your seafood as fresh and wild as you possibly can. Wild-caught seafood is typically the highest in good fats.

Avoid "pre-seasoned" or prepared seafood items. They usually contain high levels of salt and may also have MSG and other additives.

Canned, Bottled and Jarred Goods

Be sure to have plenty of olive oil, vinegars, sea salt, spices and seasonings (especially salt substitutes). Moderate salt intake is allowed, but try to cut down on salt as much as possible. You may also want organic honey, mustard, broths and stocks. Pure fruit juices are fine in small quantities, as are nut butters other than peanut butter. It is recommended to check the organic section to see if healthier versions of these types of foods are available.

Other Resources for Food

Local Farms

Due to the growing demand for healthy, high-quality foods, local farms are increasingly producing and selling organic produce and meats. Farm stands and farmers markets are excellent places to find products from these local farms.

Health Food Stores

If your grocery store has a good organic or health food section, you may be able to get everything you need there. If not, health food stores can be an excellent source for things like bulk foods, raw nuts, nut butters, nut flours, seeds and oils.

Online Resources

The Internet is an excellent resource for foods that may not be available to you locally. The popularity of the Paleo diet has spurred the online availability of Paleo-friendly products. You can order wild game, venison or just about anything else you can think of from small farms and ranches all over the country. Just be sure to do your research—not all of them produce these foods organically.

These online sources can be expensive. But if you get most of your foods at the grocery store, you can use some of the money you previously spent on fast food and vending machines to buy exotic Paleo-approved foods online.

Planning Your Paleo Diet

Knowing what to eat is half the key to success; knowing how and when to eat it is the other. The guidelines for the Paleo diet are intended to be simple, because complicated diets rarely succeed.

Don't Count Calories

Calorie counting or portioning aren't a part of the Paleo diet. The Paleo diet is a natural way of eating what your body was designed to eat; Paleolithic people often consumed a much higher number of calories and fat grams than most diets allow. Once you see the results, calorie counting will no longer be a part of your vocabulary.

On the Paleo diet, you should feel less hunger due to an increased consumption of healthy fats, lean protein and fiber. If you eat only when you're hungry, you're likely to avoid overeating without having to count calories.

The Proper Ratio of Protein to Carbs

You should try to maintain a proper ratio between your protein intake and your carb intake. The easiest way to keep this ratio in line is by looking at your menu and your plate. For all meals, at least half your plate should be protein, and half or less should be fruits, veggies, nuts and seeds.

In general, your daily diet should consist of 55 percent to 65 percent protein, 30 percent to 40 percent carbs, and 5 percent non-animal fats such as those found in nuts, seeds, avocadoes and olive oil. If you feel your energy level is dragging when you first start the diet, try increasing your carb consumption. If you find yourself snacking all day and still feeling hungry, try increasing your protein consumption.

It may take a few weeks for your body to adjust the way it converts food into energy. For the first week or two, you are likely to find yourself craving the carbs and quick energy of pasta, breads or a bowl of cereal. It's normal for your energy level to dip the first couple of weeks, but it should improve as your body begins increasingly to use protein as a source of energy.

Planning Your Daily Diet

It is recommended that you eat at least three main meals a day and several healthy snacks in between. Try to avoid going more than two hours without at least a lean protein. Snacking will keep hunger away and keep your blood sugar levels steady.

Even if you're not inclined to plan your menus in advance, many people find that doing so increases their initial chances of success. It's important to have what you need on hand so that you don't fall for an unhealthy temptation.

You will find sample meal plans in chapter 5 to inspire your planning. After a couple of weeks on the diet, you'll have a better understanding of how and when to eat and likely find it easier to create your own meal plans. To get started, here are some guidelines to help you achieve the best results.

Early Morning/Breakfast

Eat as soon as possible after you wake up, especially during your first few weeks on the Paleo diet. If you keep your evening meals protein-heavy and light on carbs, you may awaken with more energy in the morning.

Scrambled eggs and omelets are good breakfast choices if you have time to cook. If you don't have time in the morning, cold left-over meats and protein smoothies are good Paleo options.

Lunch

Lunch should include a large serving of protein, such as a meat stew, cold leftover chicken, or a salad with chicken breast or shrimp. Add some high-fiber carbs for extra fullness and energy, such as fruit with a handful of nuts.

Dinner

Your evening meals should focus primarily on protein. Most people burn less energy during the evening. Unless you work out after dinner, try to limit your carb intake. Choose low-glycemic veggies as your side dishes.

Dessert or Evening Snack

You're free to choose between a sweet treat or a little more of what you had for dinner. Fruit, unsweetened fruit ices or bars, or any of the Paleo-friendly dessert recipes included later in this book can satisfy your sweet tooth.

Snacks

Throughout your day, you should snack as frequently as possible—at least once every two to three hours. Focus on a mix of both protein and carbs for each snack. The protein will help keep you from getting hungry and the carbs will help you avoid fatigue. Eating frequently can also speed up your metabolism.

Paleo-Recommended Foods

Meats

- Eggs (from chickens, ducks or geese; do not buy egg substitutes)
- Game meats
  - Alligator
  - Bear
  - Bison (buffalo)
  - Caribou
  - Elk
  - Emu
  - Goose
  - Kangaroo
  - Muscovy duck
  - New Zealand Cervena deer
  - Ostrich
  - Pheasant
  - Quail
  - Rattlesnake
  - Reindeer
  - Squab
  - Turtle
  - Venison
  - Wild boar
  - Wild turkey
- Goat (any cut)
- Lean beef (trimmed of visible fat)
  - Chuck steak
  - Extra lean hamburger (seven percent fat or less)
  - Flank steak
  - Lean veal
  - London broil
  - Top sirloin steak
- Lean pork (trimmed of visible fat)
  - Pork chops
  - Pork loin
- Lean poultry (white meat, skin removed)
  - Chicken breast
  - Game hen breast
  - Turkey breast
- Organ meats
  - Beef, lamb, pork and chicken livers and kidneys
  - Beef, pork and lamb marrow
  - Beef, pork and lamb sweetbreads
  - Beef, pork and lamb tongues
  - Chicken and turkey gizzards and hearts
- Rabbit (any cut)

Fish

- Bass
- Bluefish
- Branzini (Mediterranean sea bass)
- Cod
- Drum
- Eel
- Flatfish
- Grouper
- Haddock
- Halibut
- Herring
- Mackerel
- Monkfish
- Mullet
- Northern pike
- Orange roughy
- Perch
- Red snapper
- Rockfish
- Salmon
- Sardine (packed in olive oil or water)
- Scrod
- Shark
- Striped bass
- Sunfish
- Swordfish
- Tilapia
- Trout
- Tuna
- Turbot
- Walleye
- Any other commercially available fish

Seafood

- Abalone
- Clam
- Crab
- Crayfish
- Lobster
- Mussel
- Oyster
- Scallop
- Shrimp

Fruits

- Apple
- Apricot
- Avocado
- Banana
- Blackberry
- Blueberry
- Boysenberry
- Cantaloupe
- Carambola
- Cherimoya
- Cherry
- Cranberry
- Gooseberry
- Grape
- Grapefruit
- Guava
- Honeydew melon
- Kiwi
- Lemon
- Lime
- Lychee
- Mango
- Nectarine
- Orange
- Papaya
- Passion fruit
- Peach
- Pear
- Persimmon
- Pineapple
- Plum
- Pomegranate
- Raspberry
- Rhubarb
- Star fruit
- Tangerine
- Watermelon

Vegetables

- Artichoke
- Asparagus
- Beet greens
- Bell pepper
- Broccoli
- Brussels sprout
- Cabbage
- Cauliflower
- Celery
- Collard greens
- Cucumber
- Dandelion greens
- Eggplant
- Endive
- Green onion
- Hot pepper (all kinds)

- Kale
- Kohlrabi
- Lettuce (except iceberg)
- Mushroom
- Mustard greens
- Onion
- Parsley
- Pumpkin
- Purslane
- Rutabaga
- Seaweed
- Spinach
- Squash (all kinds)
- Swiss chard
- Tomatillo
- Tomato
- Turnip
- Turnip greens
- Watercress
- Zucchini

Nuts, Seeds and Oils

- Almond
- Almond butter
- Brazil nut
- Cashew
- Chestnut
- Flax seed
- Hazelnut
- Macadamia nut
- Nut flour (almond and hazelnut are recommended)
- Olive oil
- Pecan
- Pine nut
- Pistachio
- Pumpkin seeds
- Sesame seeds
- Sunflower seeds
- Sesame butter or tahini (pure and raw)
- Walnut

Beverages

- Fruit juice (pure and organic, without any added sugar)
- Green tea
- Herbal tea
- Water

Other

- Carob powder
- Dried fruit without added sugar
- Fresh and dried herbs
- Frozen fruit and fruit bars without added sugar
- Raw, organic honey
- Spices and seasonings

Foods to Avoid on the Paleo Diet

Dairy

- All foods made with any dairy products
- Butter
- Cheese
- Dairy spreads
- Frozen yogurt
- Ice cream
- Ice milk
- Low-fat milk
- Nonfat dairy creamer
- Powdered milk
- Skim milk
- Whole milk
- Yogurt

Cereal Grains

- Amaranth
- Barley (barley soup, barley bread and all processed foods made with barley)
- Buckwheat

- Corn (corn on the cob, corn tortillas, corn chips, cornstarch, corn syrup)
- Millet
- Oats (steel-cut oats, rolled oats and all processed foods made with oats)
- Rice (brown rice, white rice, top ramen, rice noodles, basmati rice, rice cakes, rice flour and all processed foods made with rice)
- Rye (rye bread, rye crackers and all processed foods made with rye)
- Sorghum
- Wheat (bread, rolls, muffins, noodles, crackers, cookies, doughnuts, pancakes, waffles, pasta, spaghetti, lasagna, wheat tortillas, pizza, pita bread, flat bread and all processed foods made with wheat or wheat flour)

Legumes

- All beans (adzuki beans, black beans, broad beans, fava beans, field beans, garbanzo beans, horse beans, kidney beans, lima beans, mung beans, navy beans, pinto beans, red beans, string beans, white beans)
- Black-eyed peas
- Chickpeas
- Lentils
- Miso
- Peanuts and peanut butter
- Peas
- Snow peas
- Soybeans and all soy products, including tofu
- Sugar snap peas

Starchy Vegetables

- Cassava root
- Manioc
- Potatoes and all potato products (such as French fries and potato chips)
- Tapioca
- Yams

High-Salt Meats and Snacks

- Bacon (use the lean portions occasionally for seasoning/cooking)
- Deli meats
- Hot dogs
- Ketchup
- Kielbasa or smoked sausage
- Nearly all canned meats or and fish
- Pickled foods
- Pork rinds
- Processed meats
- Salami
- Salted nuts
- Salted spices
- Sausages
- Smoked, dried and salted fish and meat High-Salt Meats and Snacks

Other

- Canola oil
- Safflower oil
- Sugar
- Sunflower oil
- Vegetable oil

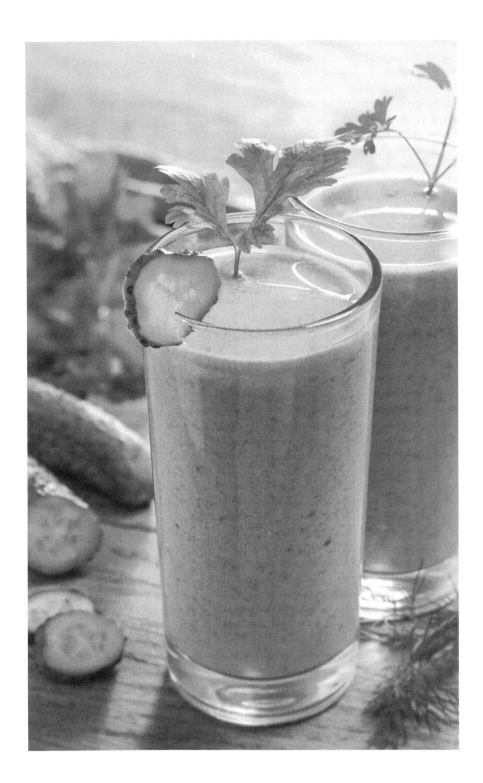

3

SET YOURSELF UP FOR SUCCESS

Diets are unlikely to be successful without the right mindset and attitude. This chapter will give you the tools to get geared up, motivated and ready to begin the Paleo diet.

Getting Your Mindset Right

Making a significant change in your habits and lifestyle is never easy. To succeed, two of the most important things you'll need are the right attitude and the right reasons for making the change.

Doing things for others is admirable, but changing your diet should be for you. If you're trying to lose weight because you want someone else's approval, you may be setting yourself up for failure; the opinions of others may not be enough to keep you on track when times get hard. Ideally, your focus should be on how you want to look, feel and improve your quality of life. The admiration from others should be merely a bonus.

The first couple of weeks of the Paleo diet are likely to require determination, willpower and commitment. For some people, the Paleo diet will require a significant change in their eating patterns.

For others, their energy level may be lower in the first few weeks. To increase your chances of success, prepare yourself for these realities.

Beginning the Paleo diet is the hardest part. Once you see and feel the results, you're likely to have all the motivation you need.

What Kind of Caveman Are You?

This quick quiz will help you understand how your lifestyle, habits and personality might affect your experience on the Paleo diet. Once you've tallied your answers, this chapter will provide some practical tips to help you succeed.

1. *Which best describes you?*

   a) I don't particularly like to cook, and I eat prepared meals or go out to eat often.

   b) I'm a pretty good cook, but I don't have much time to do so during the week.

   c) Cooking is okay, but I'm not very skilled at it.

   d) I live to cook and I consider it recreation.

2. *Are you more likely to:*

   a) Spend a lot of your free time away from home.

   b) Spend most evenings at home, tired and stressed from a busy day.

   c) Spend most evenings at home working or taking care of the kids.

   d) Entertain friends and family on weekends and during the week.

3. **Do you like to:**

   a) Try new things as long as you don't have to cook them.

   b) Keep your menu quick and simple.

   c) Stick with cooking simple basics that you know how to prepare.

   d) Try new recipes and cuisines at home.

4. **In the mornings do you:**

   a) Usually stop for breakfast on the way to work.

   b) Tend to skip breakfast and overeat later.

   c) Grab a breakfast bar or muffin at work.

   d) Always have breakfast.

If you answered A for most of the questions:

Find a few restaurants to eat at regularly that serve lean steaks, fresh seafood (not fried), and fresh vegetables and salads. Ask your server to skip the bread basket, drink plenty of water, and keep your protein-carb ratio in mind.

Be careful of skipping meals while you're away from home, especially at work. Bring deli-baked chicken, prepared salads, fresh fruits and nuts to work for handy and healthy snacks.

If you answered B for most of the questions:

Your main priority when starting the Paleo diet is going to be managing your time. Your main obstacle will be resisting the urge to grab the wrong foods because you're tired or hurried. Spend some time on the weekend preparing large batches of food for the week. This can be as simple as baking chicken legs, boiling shrimp or bagging up your own mix of nuts and dried fruit. If you have healthy meals ready to eat when you're hungry during the week, you'll be less likely to grab whatever is handy.

If you answered C for most of the questions:

Combining healthy prepared foods with some simple homemade dishes may be your best bet. An example of a healthy prepared food might be rotisserie chicken with the skin removed. A simple homemade dish could be a basic soup recipe that you make in large quantities and freeze for later, or a protein smoothie for breakfast.

If you answered D for most of the questions:

You have an advantage because you'll be able to keep meals exciting by trying lots of new ingredients and recipes. You may want to prepare a number of dishes once a week and store or freeze them to eat at work or on busier evenings. If you're cooking for your non-Paleo family in the evenings, don't try to make two meals; instead, just skip the starch or grain they're eating and pile extra proteins and veggies onto your plate.

Making the Transition

There are a number of things you can do to help ease your transition to the Paleo diet and make it enjoyable. Much like the process of preparing for a vacation, you'll want to have a plan for what you'll be doing and make sure you have everything you need. Here are some tips for making your transition smooth and simple.

Find New Food Sources

Do some research to decide where and how you'll be getting your groceries. There are great sources available both locally and online; try to identify these sources before you get started. If you're going to be using online food resources, you'll need to order ahead of time to make sure you have those foods on hand for your first week.

Spread the Word

It's a good idea to prepare the people around you for your lifestyle change. This will enable them to support you and help to avoid unintended temptation from friends who may not know that you're making a change.

In particular, it's very important to prepare roommates and family members for the changes you're making. They don't have to join you or agree with you, but they should be supportive and respectful. Talk to them before you get started and let them see that you're excited. They'll be much more likely (and able) to encourage and help you.

The First Few Weeks

Take care to avoid your dietary weak spots. Skip drinking at happy hour with your office buddies and join them for a healthy lunch instead. Go for a walk instead of sitting in front of the TV after dinner.

You might want to keep an informal journal of how you feel and what you eat during your first couple of weeks. It can be motivating and educational. As you see and feel the changes in your body, take note. These observations can help keep you on track later if you hit a rough spot.

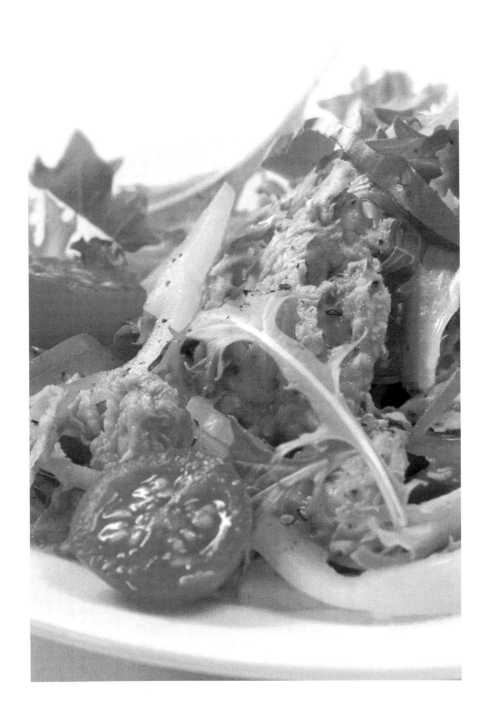

4

A WEEK OF PREPARATION—READY, SET, GO!

A week of preparation is a great way to begin your transition to the Paleo diet. Below, you'll find a list of activities that outline goals for each day of the week leading up to your Paleo transition.

Day 1: Become Your Own Best Cheerleader

Compile some of your favorite motivational quotes into a document in your computer, or write them on a piece of paper. Print or cut them out and place them in locations that you'll see every day. This might include your desk at work, your kitchen, your bathroom, or the place at home where you work out. Take the time to read and reflect on them throughout the week.

Day 2: Keep Your Vision in Front of You

Visualization is proven to be motivating when you are trying to reach a goal. Today, make yourself a vision board. You can even make two—one for home and one for your workplace. These boards can be elaborate and artistic, or a simple bulletin board or sheet of cardboard. You can even use a clipboard or dry erase board with magnets. Collect pictures that inspire you, but steer clear of pictures of fitness models and celebrities whose bodies you admire. Instead, choose pictures of things you want to do when you're fit and healthy, or even pictures of yourself when you were in better shape.

Day 3: Know Where You're Starting So You'll Know When You've Arrived

Today, you need to take stock of where you are in terms of your fitness and health. This will enable you to set realistic goals, track your progress and celebrate your success.

First, you need to take your measurements. Using a flexible tape measure, measure your chest, upper arms, waist, abdomen, hips, thighs and calves, and record the measurements. Each week, you can record the changes and see the evidence of your weight loss progress.

Next, try doing just two minutes of moderate cardio exercise. This could include jumping jacks, jumping rope or any other activity that gets you moving. Record how you feel during and after the exercise. Repeat this once a week while on the Paleo diet and notice whether your energy and fitness levels are changing.

Weigh yourself and record your starting weight, but understand that your weight is not the perfect gauge of your health. Use an online body mass index calculator (typing "BMI calculator" into a search engine will produce several free options) to calculate your body fat ratio. After starting the diet, weigh yourself and recalculate your body mass once per week. These calculations are a much better picture of how you're doing than weight alone.

Day 4: Set Your Goals

Write down goals that you would like to accomplish along with your change to a Paleo diet. Try not to go into too much detail, but avoid being too general. Establish a few weekly and/or monthly goals, such as:

I will do at least half an hour of moderate exercise three times per week.
I will cut back to two cups of caffeinated beverages per day.
I will eat breakfast every morning.
I will lose at least four pounds each month.
I will walk to work three times per week.
I will swim twenty-five laps twice per week.
I will drink at least sixty-four ounces of water each day.

Put your list of goals in a location where you can check it frequently and mark your progress. It's a good idea to change your goals every couple of weeks to keep yourself excited and moving forward.

Day 5: Make a Rewards Program for Yourself

Write down a list of rewards you will enjoy as you meet each of the goals on your list. Rewards can be as simple as buying your favorite magazine or a night out with your friends. Every success, no matter how small, should be celebrated in some way. You've earned it!

Day 6: Get Your Fill of the Forbidden

This may be your favorite day, but it isn't just for fun.

Today, go ahead and eat those favorite foods that you won't be eating on the Paleo diet. Choose the foods you love the most, whether it's pizza, ice cream or French fries. Thirty to sixty minutes after eating these foods, take a few notes on how you feel. Are you sluggish, bloated, fatigued or mentally foggy? Good. Keep those notes. Read them tomorrow when you're doing the Day 7 activity, and keep them for later if temptations arise.

Day 7: Clean House

It's time to get all the forbidden foods out of the house. That means no processed foods, sugars, legumes, dairy, processed meats, flours, bread, crackers, cookies, cakes, gravy mixes, muffins, bagels or tortillas. Here are some ideas for getting these foods out of your house.

- Donate unopened foods to a local shelter or food bank.

- Pass food boxes on to family members, friends and neighbors.

- Take canned goods to your grocery store's food donation bin or give them to the mail carrier or local firehouse if they're having a food drive.

- Take snack foods, canned fruits, unopened cereal and juices to a local day care center.

- Give unwanted items to your church or community group.

If you're living with others who will not be on the Paleo diet, then at least move their off-limits foods to separate shelves and cupboards that are less accessible and tempting to you.

Now that you've completed your preparation, you're ready to start on the Paleo diet. In the next chapter, I've laid out two weeks' worth of meal plans for you. You can use these plans exactly as they are presented, switch up some of the meals with other dishes you prefer, or just use these meal plans as a template for creating your own.

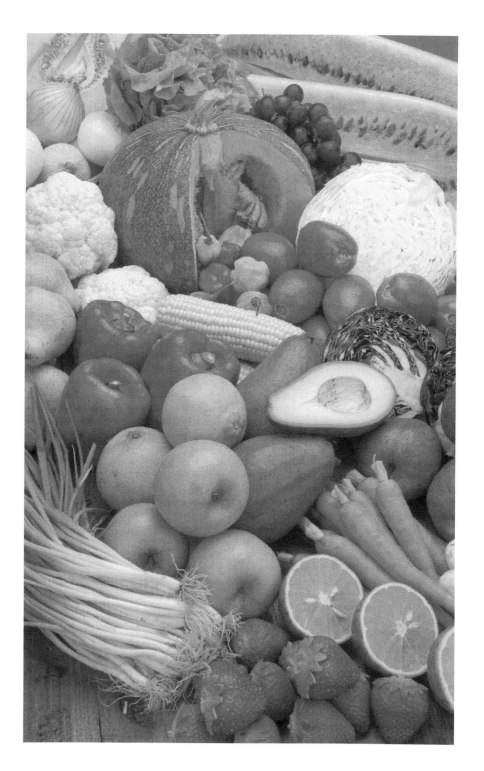

5

7-DAY MEAL PLAN

These meal plans will help you get started on the Paleo diet without having to spend too much time planning. Feel free to mix and match them a bit and try other Paleo recipes as well. Drink water at every meal, and try to drink juices only moderately.

Day 1

Breakfast
Grain-Free Pancakes

Snack
Quinoa with ground cinnamon, 1/3 cup cooked

Lunch
Sweet and Savory Chicken Salad

Dinner
Paleo Lasagna
Crispy Lemon Green Beans

Dessert
Coconut Macaroons

Day 2

Breakfast
Paleo Breakfast Burrito

Snack
Turkey jerky, ½ ounce

Lunch
Paleo Cream of Mushroom Soup
Turkey Avocado Rollups

Dinner
Zesty Meatloaf
Brussels Sprouts with Hazelnuts

Dessert
Raspberry Muffins

Day 3

Breakfast

Paleo Waffles

Snack

Blueberries, 1 cup

Lunch

Arugula, Prosciutto, and Cantaloupe Salad

Dinner

Caveman Chicken Nuggets

Paleo Fries with Herbs

Dessert

Paleo Chocolate Chip Cookies

Day 4

Breakfast

Paleo Huevos Rancheros

Snack

Unsweetened applesauce, 1 cup

Lunch

Hearty Paleo Stew

Dinner

Nectarine and Onion Pork Chops

Roasted Broccoli

Dessert

Banana Bread

Day 5

Breakfast
Paleo Granola

Snack
Oven-roasted deli turkey, 2 slices

Lunch
Tuna Salad with a Twist

Dinner
Grilled Lamb Chops
Simple Grilled Asparagus

Dessert
Berry Tart

Day 6

Breakfast
Paleo Muffins

Snack
Hummus, 4 tablespoons with carrot sticks

Lunch
Walnut and Beet Salad
Crab-Stuffed Mushrooms

Dinner
Pulled Pork with Homemade Barbecue Sauce
Roasted Sweet Potatoes with Rosemary

Dessert
Poached Pears

Day 7

Breakfast

Zesty Breakfast Salad

Snack

Mandarin oranges, 1 snack cup

Lunch

Spicy Southwestern Chicken Soup

Dinner

Lemon and Garlic Roasted Chicken

Kale with Walnuts and Cranberries

Dessert

Primal Brownies

6

BREAKFASTS

Grain-Free Pancakes

Nut butter and eggs make fine substitutes for flour in these pancakes. The pancakes cook up light, flavorful and slightly creamy, and with 9.5 grams of protein per serving, they'll keep you full for hours. Drizzle them with a bit of honey for a sweet taste if necessary, but remember to watch your sugar intake—especially for breakfast.

- 4 ripe bananas
- 4 large eggs
- ½ cup nut butter
- Freshly ground black pepper, to taste
- 2 teaspoons olive or coconut oil

Place the bananas in a large bowl and mash them with a fork until smooth.

Beat the eggs in a separate bowl until frothy. Add them to the bananas.

Add the nut butter and mix well until creamy and smooth. Season with freshly ground black pepper to taste.

Heat the olive oil in a skillet or on a griddle. Pour ¼ cup pancake batter for each pancake onto the griddle or skillet.

Cook pancakes for 2 minutes and then flip with a spatula. Cook 2 minutes on the other side, or until the pancakes are golden brown.

Serves 4

Zesty Breakfast Salad

Salad for breakfast? Sure! This fruit and nut salad has a citrus dressing that will wake up your taste buds and get you ready for the day. Hard-boiled eggs and bacon add protein to keep you full for hours.

Salad:
- 2 cups baby spinach
- 1 large egg, hard-boiled and sliced into ½-inch chunks
- 1 strip uncured, nitrate-free bacon, cooked and crumbled
- 1 Clementine orange, peeled and quartered
- ½ cup dried cranberries or cherries
- ½ cup macadamia nuts, black walnuts, or pecans
- Freshly ground black pepper, to taste

Dressing:
- 1 tablespoon honey
- 1 teaspoon dry mustard
- ¼ cup red wine vinegar
- Juice of one orange
- 1 teaspoon onion, finely minced
- 1 cup olive oil
- Zest of 1 orange

In a medium non-stick skillet, heat the oil over medium heat. Add the onion and bell pepper and cook until soft. Add the sausage and eggs and stir continuously until eggs are cooked through. Season with freshly ground black pepper.

To serve, divide between plates and top with avocado and salsa.

Serves 2

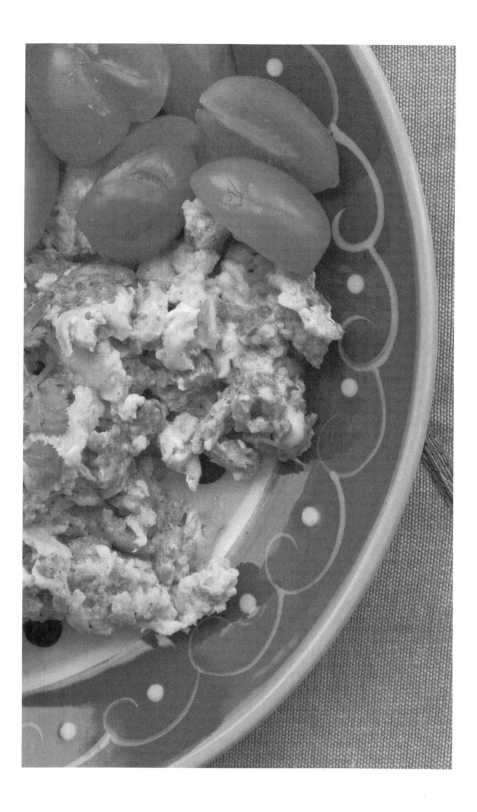

Mexican Veggie Scramble

Loaded with veggies and high-protein eggs, this dish is filling and easy to make, but also delicious. Garnish with avocado and your favorite salsa for a south-of-the-border meal you won't forget. Think you'll miss the cheese? You may be surprised.

- 1 tablespoon olive or coconut oil
- ½ small onion, chopped
- ½ green bell pepper, diced
- ½ pound minimally processed chorizo sausage, cooked and crumbled
- 4 large eggs, beaten
- Freshly ground black pepper, to taste
- Sliced avocado, for garnish
- Prepared salsa, for garnish

In a medium non-stick skillet, heat the oil over medium heat. Add the onion and bell pepper and cook until soft. Add the sausage and eggs and stir continuously until eggs are cooked through. Season with freshly ground black pepper.

To serve, divide between plates and top with avocado and salsa.

Serves 2

Paleo Breakfast Burrito

If you're craving a breakfast burrito, you'll love this Paleo-adapted recipe. Instead of a tortilla filled with eggs and meat, the eggs become the tortilla, leaving you with the same flavors rolled up into a tasty, easy to eat breakfast that will leave you full for hours. For best results, use a medium-sized skillet so that your eggs are super thin and easy to wrap. You'll never miss out on the high-carb tortilla!

- ¼ pound grass-fed ground beef
- 1 teaspoon cumin
- 1 teaspoon garlic powder
- 1 teaspoon onion powder
- 3 large eggs, beaten
- 1 tablespoon olive or coconut oil
- ½ small red onion, finely chopped
- Freshly ground black pepper, to taste
- Fresh cilantro, chopped, for garnish
- Prepared salsa for serving

Brown the beef in a skillet over medium heat. Once the meat is no longer pink, add the onion and season with the cumin, garlic powder, and onion powder. Set aside.

Whisk eggs in a small mixing bowl. Heat oil in a medium skillet over medium-low heat. Add the eggs in a thin, even layer and cook for about 6 minutes. Carefully flip the eggs over and continue cooking until done. Season with freshly ground black pepper. Carefully slide the eggs onto a plate. Top with the seasoned meat, cilantro, and salsa.

Serves 1

High-Protein Frittata

This is an easy breakfast dish that is loaded with protein. You can customize it to your liking, so use whatever veggies you like or have in your fridge. This is a great way to use up leftovers.

- 1 tablespoon olive or coconut oil
- ½ small onion, chopped
- ½ cup mushrooms, sliced
- 2 cups baby spinach leaves
- 8 large eggs
- Freshly ground black pepper, to taste
- 4 strips of uncured, nitrate-free bacon, cooked and crumbled

Preheat oven to 350 degrees F. Heat a large ovenproof skillet over medium heat and add the oil and vegetables. Sauté until tender. Remove from skillet and set aside.

Beat eggs in a large bowl and add the cooked vegetables. Season with freshly ground black pepper. Pour mixture into the skillet and put in the oven. Bake for 12 to 15 minutes or until eggs are firm to the touch.

Top with crumbled bacon and serve immediately.

Serves 4

Eggs Benedict Paleo Style

While this might not be the traditional version of eggs Benedict, you'll love this grain-free version that is as good for you as it tastes. Once you try it, you'll never want to go back to the old version again!

- ½ medium avocado
- 2 tablespoons lemon juice
- 1 clove garlic
- 1 large egg
- 1 tomato slice
- 2 slices uncured, nitrate-free bacon, cooked and crumbled
- Freshly ground black pepper, to taste

Put the avocado, lemon juice, and garlic in a food processor and process until smooth and creamy.

Poach the egg in a pot of simmering water until done, about 4 minutes.

To serve, place the egg on top of the tomato slice and top with the avocado sauce and bacon. Season with freshly ground black pepper.

Serves 1

Egg Casserole for One

Sometimes you are in the mood for a delicious breakfast casserole filled with eggs, veggies, and breakfast meats, but you don't have the time or need for a full-fledged kitchen marathon. If this is the case, this recipe fits the bill. It's fast, easy, and doesn't leave you with leftovers you can't eat. For two, simply double the recipe and divide between two ramekins, or use a casserole dish if you're serving more than one. Either way, you'll love it!

- 2 large eggs
- 2 broccoli florets, finely chopped
- ¼ small zucchini, chopped
- ¼ small onion, chopped
- 5 spinach leaves, chopped
- 2 slices uncured, nitrate-free bacon, cooked and crumbled
- 1 tablespoon olive or coconut oil
- Freshly ground black pepper, to taste

Preheat oven to 350 degrees F. Beat eggs in a small bowl and mix in the veggies and bacon. Season with freshly ground black pepper.

Grease a single-serve ramekin with oil and pour the egg mixture in. Bake for 15 to 20 minutes until the top is lightly browned. Serve immediately.

Serves 1

Scrambled Eggs with Lox

Traditionally, lox is served with high-carb bagels and cream cheese. While these may taste good, neither fits in a Paleo lifestyle. This version uses high-protein eggs and sliced tomatoes for a healthier version that you'll find just as tasty as the original. Smoked whitefish works well here too for a change of pace once in a while.

- 1 tablespoon olive or coconut oil
- ½ small red onion, diced
- 3 large eggs
- 2 ounces smoked salmon, chopped
- Freshly ground black pepper, to taste
- 1 large tomato, sliced
- 1 teaspoon capers
- 1 tablespoon fresh parsley, chopped

Heat oil in a medium skillet and add the onions. Cook until soft.

Beat the eggs in a small bowl and add the salmon. Season with freshly ground black pepper. Pour egg mixture over onions and scramble until cooked through.

To serve, top the tomato slices with the eggs and garnish with capers and parsley.

Serves 1

Chicken with Sweet Potato Hash Browns

It's hard to find a breakfast on the Paleo plan that doesn't include eggs, but this is one. You can serve it with eggs if you'd like, of course, but this dish stands on its own pretty well. Dark-meat chicken works nicely here, but use whatever you have on hand—it will still be delicious. The sweet potatoes make an excellent substitute for traditional greasy and high-carb hash brown potatoes.

- 2 sweet potatoes, peeled and diced into small pieces
- 2 tablespoons olive oil
- ½ small onion, diced
- 4 chicken thighs, cooked, meat pulled off bones and chopped or shredded
- 1 teaspoon each, dried thyme and oregano
- Freshly ground black pepper, to taste

Either in a microwave or steamer, steam sweet potatoes until tender and easily pierced with a fork. Divide in half and mash one half with a fork or potato masher.

In a large skillet, heat oil over medium-high heat. Add onion and cook until tender. Add chicken and spices, except pepper, and combine.

Add both sweet potato mixtures to the pan and combine the mixture thoroughly. Season with freshly ground black pepper.

Continue cooking until browned on the bottom, then flip to cook the other side until browned. Break up into small pieces and serve.

Serves 4

Paleo Muffins

There's a reason why muffins are popular breakfast items: They're easy to grab and go. Unfortunately, what you gain in convenience, you usually give up in health content. Not so with these muffins. Loaded with veggies, they are easy to whip up and you can keep them around for those mornings when you just need something you can grab as you're headed out the door. No more worrying about indulging in high-carb muffins when you've got this high-protein version on hand.

- 1 teaspoon olive or coconut oil
- ½ medium onion, chopped
- 1 cup broccoli, finely chopped
- ½ green bell pepper, diced
- ½ red bell pepper, diced
- 8 large eggs
- Freshly ground black pepper, to taste

Preheat oven to 400 degrees F. Grease a muffin tin with oil. Mix veggies in a large bowl and divide equally among muffin tins.

Beat eggs in a large bowl. Season with freshly ground black pepper. Pour mixture over veggies in the muffin pan.

Bake for 15 to 20 minutes, or until tops are browned. Loosen with a knife around the edges and cool before serving.

Makes 1 dozen

Paleo Huevos Rancheros

This popular egg dish is usually served with corn tortillas and beans, but once you try this version, you'll be surprised by how tasty it can be without those high-carb additions. You don't need those energy-sucking carbs for breakfast! This makes a fabulous brunch option as well.

- 1 tablespoon olive or coconut oil
- 2 cloves garlic, minced
- 1 red bell pepper, chopped
- ½ small onion, diced
- 1 jalapeño pepper, minced
- 2 large eggs
- Freshly ground black pepper, to taste
- ½ cup prepared salsa
- ½ medium avocado, sliced

Heat oil in a medium skillet over medium heat. Add the garlic, bell pepper, onion, and jalapeño pepper, and sauté until soft. Add the eggs and cook until the whites are cooked through. Season with freshly ground black pepper.

To serve, top the eggs and veggies with salsa and avocado. Serve immediately.

Serves 1

Classic French Omelet

Some dishes need to be adapted to fit the Paleo lifestyle, but a French omelet is one that fits perfectly. Well, almost perfectly. Most French omelets have cheese in them. If you try it without, however, you may find it's just as enjoyable. It may take practice to get the perfect visual effect, but the results are so delicious that you won't mind the practice it takes to get there.

- 3 large eggs
- 1 tablespoon olive or coconut oil
- 2 tablespoons chopped fresh herbs of your choice
- Freshly ground black pepper, to taste
- 2 slices minimally processed ham

Beat eggs in a bowl and set aside. Heat a non-stick skillet over medium heat and add the oil.

Add eggs, followed by herbs. Season with freshly ground black pepper. Cook for 1 minute and add the ham to the center. Once the eggs begin to cook, fold both sides toward the center.

Slide onto a plate and serve with extra ham slices and herbs for garnish.

Serves 1

Paleo Western Omelet

Eggs are classics when it comes to Paleo diet recipes, and for good reason. High in protein as well as vitamins and minerals, they are what some would call a "super food." Even better, they are ridiculously easy to cook. This recipe has been modified just a bit to fit the Paleo diet, but you won't notice the difference, as it's super delicious.

- 3 large eggs
- 1 tablespoon olive oil
- 2 ounces minimally processed, thick-cut ham
- ¼ cup chopped bell pepper
- ¼ cup onion, chopped
- ½ cup spinach, finely chopped
- Freshly ground black pepper, to taste

Beat the eggs until frothy.

Add oil to a non-stick omelet pan and heat over medium heat. Add eggs. As they start to set, add the ham and veggies, spreading evenly throughout.

Fold over and finish cooking. Season with freshly ground black pepper. When eggs are thoroughly cooked, slide onto a plate and serve.

Serves 1

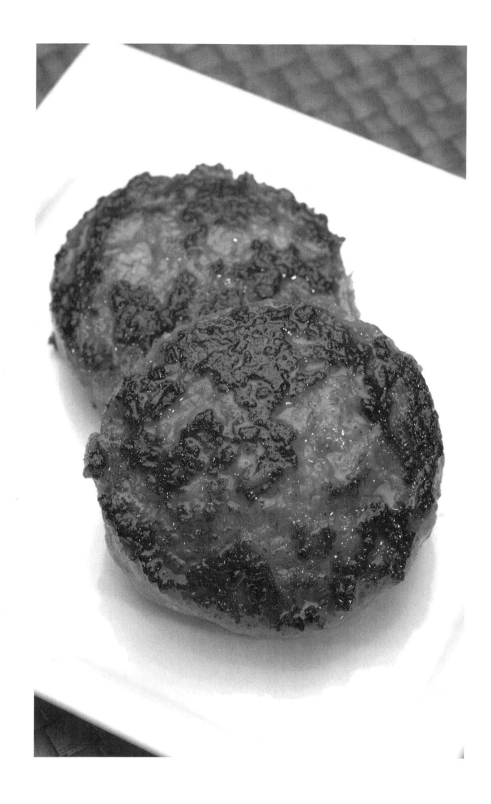

Homemade Breakfast Patties

While sausage technically fits on the Paleo diet, it can be hard to find a variety that isn't laced with added chemicals and fillers. Since you want to avoid these types of ingredients, making your own sausage is the best route to take. It's also one that is not nearly as difficult as it may sound, and the results are worth it. Feel free to adjust your seasonings to suit your personal tastes.

- 1 pound ground pork
- 1 teaspoon garlic powder
- 1 teaspoon paprika
- ½ teaspoon ground sage
- 1 teaspoon fennel seeds
- ¼ teaspoon cayenne pepper
- ¼ teaspoon white pepper
- 2 tablespoons olive or coconut oil
- Freshly ground black pepper, to taste

Using your hands, combine the pork with the seasonings in a large bowl until well combined.

Form into 8 to 10 patties. Heat a medium skillet over medium heat and add the oil. Fry the sausage patties until golden brown on both sides (about 4 minutes per side), making sure the inside is no longer pink. Season with freshly ground black pepper.

Serve immediately.

Serves 4

Caveman French Toast

While you might think the bread is the most important ingredient in French toast, you should try this recipe anyway. It's just eggs with French toast seasonings, and it really is quite delicious. Once you try it, it will probably become one of your favorite Paleo diet recipes. Make sure you use only real maple syrup, and not too much!

- 4 large eggs
- 1 tablespoon water
- 1 teaspoon vanilla extract
- 1 teaspoon cinnamon
- Pinch of nutmeg
- 1 tablespoon coconut oil
- Pure maple syrup for drizzling

In a small bowl, beat the eggs and water together until frothy. Add vanilla, cinnamon, and nutmeg.

Heat a non-stick omelet pan on medium-high heat. When hot, add coconut oil and swirl pan to coat.

Add half the egg mixture to the pan and let it cook through before flipping. Cook until browned on both sides.

Serves 2

Italian Frittata

Casseroles are comfort foods, and this one is no exception. A delicious recipe for a brunch, or even a lazy Sunday breakfast, this is one of the best Paleo recipes you'll find.

- 2 tablespoons olive oil
- 1 small onion, diced
- 2 cloves garlic, minced
- 1 zucchini, diced
- 1 pound spinach, coarsely chopped
- 12 cherry tomatoes, quartered
- ½ cup black olives
- Freshly ground black pepper, to taste
- 12 large eggs

Preheat oven to 375 degrees F.

In a large sauté pan, heat the oil over medium-high heat. Add the onions and garlic and cook until soft. Add the zucchini and continue cooking for a couple more minutes. Add spinach, combine and cook until wilted. Remove pan from heat and add the tomatoes and olives. Season with freshly ground black pepper.

In a large bowl, whisk the eggs until frothy.

Lightly brush the bottom of an 8 x 13-inch casserole dish with oil. Add the veggies to the dish. Pour over the egg mixture and stir to combine.

Bake for an hour until the top is browned and the center is cooked through. Slice into squares and serve.

Serves 6

Paleo Granola

Traditional granola doesn't work on the Paleo plan: It's loaded with oats, sugar, and other processed or high-carb ingredients. If you want something other than eggs for breakfast, this version fits the bill. It's got nuts, fruit, and coconut and is easy to prepare and store for a quick snack as well.

- 1 cup raw pecans
- 1 cup raw sunflower seeds
- 1 cup raw walnuts
- 1 cup raw sliced almonds
- 1 cup raw pumpkin seeds
- 1 cup unsweetened coconut, shredded
- 1 cup Medjool dates, chopped
- 1 cup raisins

Soak nuts and seeds overnight in warm water, about 10 hours. Drain well.

Spread the nuts and seeds on a baking sheet in an even layer. Set oven to the lowest temperature possible and put the baking sheet in the oven door open, dehydrate nuts for 10 hours. Allow to cool completely.

Chop nuts and seeds and combine with the coconut, dates, and raisins. Serve either as a snack or with unsweetened almond milk as a breakfast cereal.

Serves 8

Paleo Spinach Quiche

Traditional quiche is usually loaded with cheese, but you won't miss it in this flavorful recipe. It's a great dish to make the night before, especially if you already have the oven on for dinner.

- 1 teaspoon olive oil, plus more for greasing the pan
- 1 cup chopped fresh spinach
- ½ cup chopped red onion
- ½ teaspoon salt
- ½ teaspoon freshly ground black pepper
- ½ teaspoon ground nutmeg
- 8 large eggs, beaten
- ½ cup plain almond milk

Preheat oven to 350 degrees F. Grease a 9-inch glass pie plate.

In a small skillet, heat the olive oil over medium heat, and sauté the spinach, onion, salt, pepper, and nutmeg for about 5 minutes, or just until the onions are translucent.

Stir the eggs and almond milk together in a small bowl. Add the spinach mixture, stir, and pour into the pie plate.

Bake the quiche on the middle oven rack for 30 to 40 minutes, or until the center is completely set. Serve warm or at room temperature.

Serves 4 to 6

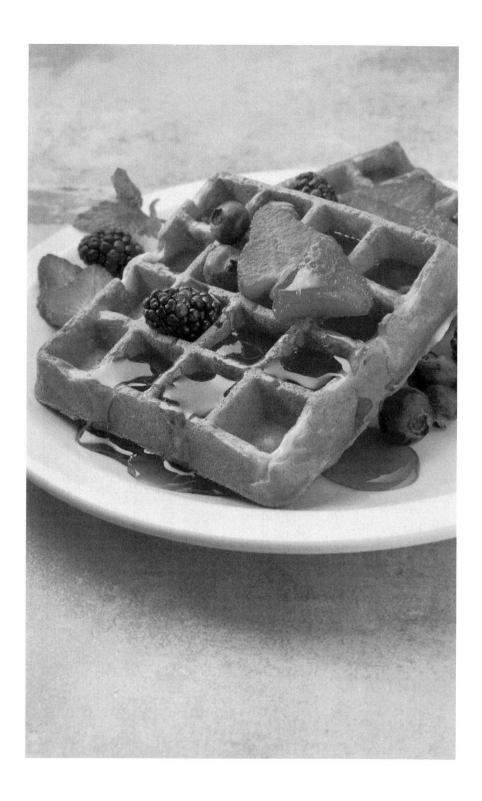

Paleo Waffles

While this isn't something you want to eat everyday, the use of coconut flour in these waffles allows you to indulge once in a while, for a special occasion, or just a weekend treat.

- ¼ cup coconut flour
- 4 large eggs
- 1 tablespoon coconut milk
- 1 tablespoon cinnamon
- ¼ teaspoon nutmeg
- ¼ teaspoon baking soda
- Pure maple syrup

Preheat a waffle iron. Blend all ingredients in a blender or by hand in a bowl. Pour batter in the center of the waffle iron, covering the entire surface area.

Cook until waffles release from the iron. Serve immediately with maple syrup.

Serves 2

Banana-Berry Pancakes

*These pancakes get their natural sweetness from berries and bananas.
The recipe calls for raspberries, but you can substitute any type of berry.
Berries are a great choice for the Paleo diet. They're high in antioxidants
and add intense flavor and sweetness to any dish.*

- 6 egg whites, lightly beaten
- 2 bananas, mashed
- ⅓ cup raspberries, mashed
- 2 tablespoons almond butter
- ¼ teaspoon cinnamon

Spray a skillet or griddle with cooking spray. In a large bowl, mix the
egg whites, bananas, raspberries, and almond butter until smooth.

Pour the batter into the skillet using ½ cup for each pancake. Wait 2
to 3 minutes before flipping the pancakes. Cook an additional 2 to
3 minutes until golden brown. Serve with a sprinkling of cinnamon
and/or fresh fruit.

Serves 2

7

SOUPS, SALADS, AND DRESSINGS

Creamy Asparagus Soup

Soups are surprisingly satisfying and are usually nutrient dense as well. Asparagus has a fresh, slightly acerbic taste that pairs well with the cream in this soup. Asparagus is available year-round, although it's at its best in the spring. Look for bright green stalks with closed tips. Open tips indicate the asparagus is old.

- 2 tablespoons olive or coconut oil
- ¼ cup finely chopped shallots
- 1 pound asparagus, steamed
- Freshly ground black pepper, to taste
- 2 cups chicken stock, preferably homemade
- 1 cup full-fat coconut milk
- 1 tablespoon organic white wine

Heat the oil in a large saucepan. Sauté the shallots for 5 minutes, or until tender. Place the shallots and the steamed asparagus in a blender or food processor and puree until smooth. Season with freshly ground black pepper.

Transfer the asparagus puree back to the saucepan. Add the remaining ingredients and heat to a simmer. Simmer for 20 minutes and serve.

Serves 4

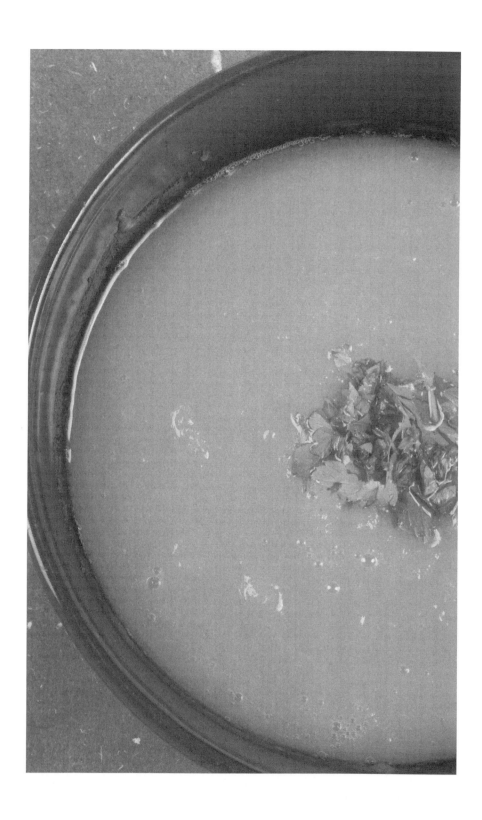

Classic Pumpkin Soup

Classic and simple, this recipe combines sweet potatoes and pumpkin to create a delicious and somewhat unusual soup. Don't let the simplicity of the ingredients fool you — it is bursting with flavor and makes a great soup for a lazy fall afternoon. Add a touch of cinnamon or nutmeg for a little extra spice.

- 2 tablespoons olive or coconut oil
- 1 onion, chopped
- 1 garlic minced
- 1½ pounds pumpkin flesh, chopped roughly
- 2 medium sweet potatoes, peeled and roughly chopped
- Freshly ground black pepper, to taste
- 4 cups chicken stock
- 1 cup canned coconut milk

Add the cooking oil to a large pot and simmer the onions in it until they are soft. Add garlic and simmer until you begin to smell the aroma.

Add chopped pumpkin and sweet potatoes, cook for a few minutes. Season with freshly ground black pepper.

Add the stock. Bring to a boil and let simmer for approximately 25 minutes, or until the sweet potatoes and pumpkin are tender.

Stir in the coconut milk.

Serve with an extra dash of coconut milk on top.

Serves 4

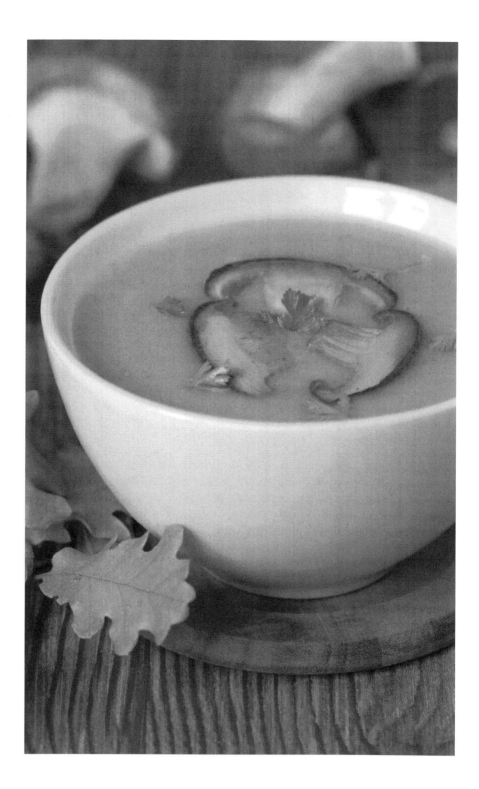

Paleo Cream of Mushroom Soup

This delicious creamed soup gets it's texture from avocado. It's a filling and flavorful soup that makes a great starter course to a Paleo dinner, but it can also make a light meal in itself when served with a green salad.

- 2 ripe avocados
- Juice of 1 lemon
- 2 cloves garlic, minced
- 2 cups water
- 1 tablespoon olive or coconut oil
- 1 cup mushrooms, sliced
- 1 red bell pepper, diced
- ½ small onion, diced
- 2 tomatoes, seeded and diced
- Fresh chopped basil, for garnish
- Freshly ground black pepper, to taste

In a food processor, blend avocado, lemon juice, garlic, and 2 cups water. Set aside.

Meanwhile, heat a medium saucepan with tall sides over medium-high heat. Add the oil.

Sauté mushrooms, bell pepper, onion, and tomatoes until they begin to soften.

Add the blended avocado mixture and simmer until warmed through. Season with basil and freshly ground black pepper. Serve immediately.

Serves 4

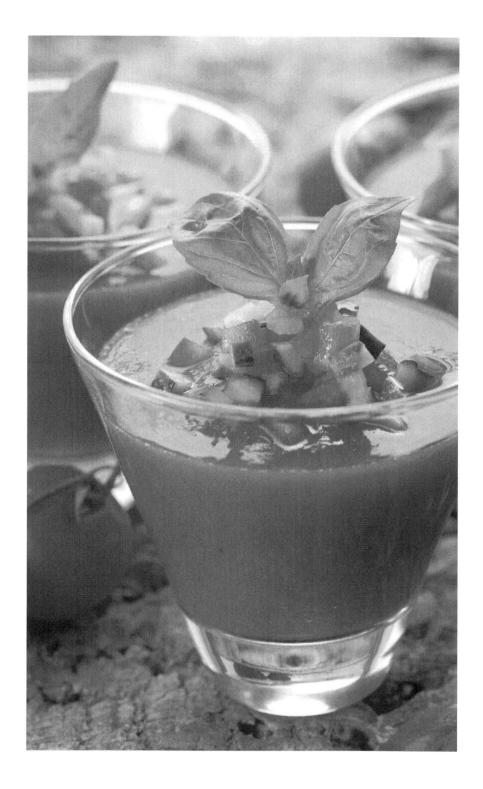

Classic Gazpacho

If you've never had gazpacho, you don't know what you're missing. Essentially a cold soup, it's a refreshing starter in the heat of summer when you don't want something hot, but can't stand to eat another salad. This classic tomato version is easy, refreshing, and sure to become a household staple.

- 4 large, ripe tomatoes, roughly chopped
- 1 small onion, chopped
- 1 medium cucumber, peeled and chopped
- 1 small bunch fresh parsley
- 1 clove garlic, chopped
- Juice of 1 lemon
- 1 cup ice-cold water
- Freshly ground black pepper, to taste

Put all ingredients in a blender or food processor and process until vegetables are finely chopped. If you would like a pureed soup, continue blending until desired consistency. Season with freshly ground black pepper.

Chill for at least 1 hour and serve cold.

Serves 4

Hearty Paleo Stew

Is there anything more satisfying than a big bowl of beef stew? This recipe is modified (although just slightly) to fit right in with the plan so you won't miss a beat. If you don't have turnips, you can just as easily substitute sweet potatoes.

- 4 slices uncured, nitrate-free bacon, diced
- 4 to 6 pounds grass-fed beef roast, cubed
- 1 small onion, finely chopped
- 2 garlic cloves, minced
- 2 large carrots, diced
- 2 turnips, diced
- 1 cup tomatoes, diced
- 1 teaspoon dried thyme
- Freshly ground black pepper, to taste
- 1 to 2 cups beef or chicken stock

Heat a large stockpot and add bacon. Cook until almost crisp, and add the cubed beef. Sear on all sides until golden brown.

Add onion and garlic, cook until both are soft, add carrots, turnips, tomatoes, and thyme. Simmer 5 minutes. Season with freshly ground black pepper.

Add stock and bring to a boil. Reduce heat and simmer 4 to 5 hours on low heat, or until beef is melt-in-your-mouth tender, and serve.

Serves 4 to 6

Spicy Southwestern Chicken Soup

Every culture has its version of chicken soup—all hearty and soul satisfying. And Grandma was right—chicken soup contains anti-inflammatory properties that can relieve cold symptoms, according to the University of Nebraska Medical Center. This chicken soup is perfect for the Paleo diet. It's chock-full of chicken (for protein) and tasty vegetables.

- 2 tablespoons olive or coconut oil
- ½ cup onion, chopped
- ½ cup red bell pepper, chopped
- ½ cup zucchini, chopped
- 1 teaspoon garlic, minced
- 1 (8-ounce) can roasted, chopped green chilies
- 1 (14-ounce) can diced tomatoes with chilies
- 4 cups chicken stock
- 2 cups cooked chicken, shredded
- 2 teaspoons cumin
- 2 teaspoons chili powder
- ½ teaspoon cayenne pepper
- Freshly ground black pepper, to taste

Heat the oil in a large stockpot. Add the onions, bell pepper, zucchini, and garlic and cook until tender.

Add the remaining ingredients and heat to simmering. Season with freshly ground black pepper. Simmer for 30 minutes and serve.

Serves 4

Veggie Soup with a Kick

While this is not a vegetarian recipe, it is loaded with filling, high-fiber vegetables and lots of protein. Fresh vegetables work well here, and you can substitute whatever you have or like—just be sure to stay away from starchy vegetables like white potatoes and corn.

- 4 slices uncured, nitrate-free, thick-cut bacon, diced
- 1 onion, diced
- 1 green bell pepper, diced
- 2 medium carrots, diced
- 2 zucchini, diced
- ½ head cabbage, shredded
- 1 pound grass-fed ground beef
- 1 cup canned tomatoes with juice
- 1 tablespoon chili powder
- ½ teaspoon cayenne pepper
- 2 cups chicken or beef stock
- Freshly ground black pepper, to taste

Heat a large pot or Dutch oven over medium-high heat. Add the bacon and cook until crisp.

Add the onion and bell pepper and cook until softened.

Add carrots, zucchini, and cabbage, cooking until carrots are slightly tender, approximately 5 minutes.

Add ground beef and cook until browned, and then add tomatoes and seasonings, followed by stock. Bring to a boil.

Reduce heat and simmer until carrots and beef are cooked through. Season with freshly ground black pepper. Serve piping hot.

Serves 6

Velvety Squash Soup

Apples and butternut squash complement each other perfectly and are widely available in the fall. Try roasting the two together for a dinner side dish, and save enough to make this tasty soup. Butternut squash stores well in a cool pantry, but you can also freeze cubed butternut squash for later use.

- 2 tablespoons olive or coconut oil
- 2 cups butternut squash, peeled and cubed
- 1 cup apples, peeled, cored, and quartered
- ½ cup shallots
- 4 cups chicken stock
- ½ cup full-fat coconut milk
- ½ teaspoon thyme
- Freshly ground black pepper, to taste
- 2 strips uncured, nitrate-free bacon, cooked and crumbled

Preheat oven to 450 degrees F. Heat the oil in the microwave. Spread the butternut squash, apples, and shallots on a baking sheet. Add the olive or coconut oil and toss to coat. Roast for 15 to 25 minutes, or until tender, stirring frequently so the shallots don't burn.

Transfer the squash, shallots, and apples to a blender or food processor and puree until smooth. Pour the mixture into a stockpot and add the stock, coconut milk, and thyme. Season with freshly ground black pepper. Simmer for 20 minutes. Top with crumbled bacon.

Serve piping hot.

Serves 6

Sweet and Savory Chicken Salad

A great combination of chicken mixed with fruits and vegetables makes this salad a unique and tasty treat. Unlike most chicken salads, the grouping of avocado and mayonnaise adds a flavorful side while the apples, grapes, and cranberries add a distinctly sweet side. Top with walnuts and celery to add an extra-crunchy texture.

- 4 boneless, skinless chicken breasts, cooked and shredded
- ½ cup dried cranberries
- 1 cup celery, chopped
- ¾ cup green grapes, halved
- ½ cup walnuts, chopped
- 1 avocado, peeled, pitted and diced
- 1 apple, peeled, cored and chopped
- 1 cup olive-oil mayonnaise
- Juice of 1 lemon
- Freshly ground black pepper, to taste

Combine the chicken, cranberries, celery, grapes, walnuts, avocado, and apple in a large bowl and mix well.

In a separate bowl, combine the mayonnaise with the lemon juice and whisk.

Add the dressing into the large bowl with the chicken mixture and toss until all are coated well in the dressing. Season with freshly ground black pepper. Serve chilled.

Serves 4

Tuna Salad with a Twist

Tuna is the perfect high-protein food for those following the Paleo diet. Green onions, jalapeños, ginger, and red chili flakes definitely give this salad a zesty bite. Served on a bed of lettuce, this dish makes for a satisfying meal.

- 2 cans white albacore tuna
- 1 cup green olives, chopped
- 2 green onions, chopped
- 1 jalapeño pepper, finely chopped
- 3 tablespoons capers, rinsed
- 1 tablespoon pickled ginger, chopped
- ½ teaspoon red chili flakes
- Juice of 1 lemon
- Juice of 1 lime
- 1 tablespoon olive oil
- 1 head butter lettuce or mixed greens
- 1 avocado, pitted and sliced
- Freshly ground black pepper, to taste

In a mixing bowl, combine all of the ingredients except the lettuce and avocado. Season with freshly ground black pepper.

Divide the lettuce between two chilled plates and place half the tuna mixture onto each. Arrange half of the avocado onto each salad and serve immediately.

Serves 2

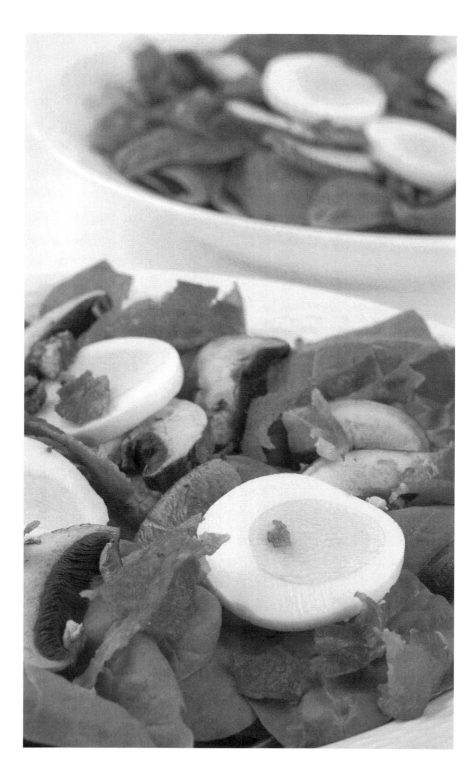

Bacon and Spinach Salad

Bacon goes with everything but is especially nice with spinach. The walnuts and hard-boiled eggs add a nice variety of flavors and textures to this dish, making this a great salad for a full meal. You can also add a protein such as grilled chicken breast or a piece of broiled fish for a nice flavor profile.

- 1 pound fresh spinach, washed, drained, and torn into bite-sized pieces
- 1 can sliced water chestnuts, drained
- 1 pound fresh mushrooms, thinly sliced
- Freshly ground black pepper, to taste

- 6 slices uncured, nitrate-free bacon, cooked and crumbled
- ½ cup walnuts, chopped and toasted
- 4 large eggs, hard-boiled and sliced

Combine the spinach with the water chestnuts and mushrooms. Season with freshly ground black pepper. Divide between two plates.

Top with crumbled bacon, walnuts, and sliced eggs. Serve immediately.

Serves 2

Easy Greek Salad

Avocado, sun-dried tomatoes, and artichoke, along with crunchy onion and bell peppers, create a satisfying salad loaded with flavor — a nice variation on a classic Greek salad. For best results, use the freshest vegetables you can get your hands on.

- 2 tablespoons balsamic vinegar
- 3 tablespoons olive oil
- 1 teaspoon Greek seasoning
- 1 ripe avocado
- 1 green bell pepper, sliced
- ¼ medium red onion, sliced
- 1 cup black olives, pitted and cut in half
- 2 tomatoes, cut into bite-sized pieces
- ½ cucumber, halved and sliced
- ⅛ cup sun-dried tomatoes packed in olive oil
- ⅛ cup artichoke hearts
- Freshly ground black pepper, to taste

Whisk together the balsamic vinegar, olive oil, and Greek seasoning.

Combine the rest of the ingredients with the dressing. Season with freshly ground black pepper.

Let chill covered in the refrigerator for 30 minutes before serving.

Serves 2

Arugula, Prosciutto, and Cantaloupe Salad

Prosciutto is the perfect match to melon, bringing out the salty, savory flavor of the ham and the sweetness of the cantaloupe. The arugula adds a nice spicy contrast and the walnuts add a bit of crunch. This salad is best in the summer when you can get a fresh melon that is picked at the perfect time.

- 4 cups arugula, loosely packed
- 6 slices good quality prosciutto, cut into ½-inch strips
- ½ cantaloupe, seeds and rind removed, cut into ½-inch cubes
- 1 cup walnuts, roughly chopped
- Freshly ground black pepper, to taste
- Olive oil, to taste

Divide the arugula among four plates.

Top the arugula with prosciutto, cantaloupe, and walnuts. Season with freshly ground black pepper.

Drizzle a little olive oil over each salad.

Serves 4

Crab and Mango Salad

Crab is a good source of protein and omega-3 fatty acids. The mango adds a nice sweet-and-sour component to the salad. One bite of this salad and you'll think you're on an island in the Caribbean—especially if you can eat it outside on a nice sunny day.

- 4 cups mixed baby greens
- ¼ cup fresh cooked crabmeat, picked over for shells
- 1 mangos, peeled and diced
- ½ cucumber, peeled and sliced thin
- Juice from 2 limes
- 1 tablespoon fresh mint, roughly chopped
- 2 teaspoons olive oil
- Freshly ground black pepper, to taste

Divide the mixed lettuce between two plates.

Toss the remaining ingredients together in a bowl. Season with freshly ground black pepper.

Divide the crab salad between the two plates, heaping it in the center of the lettuce.

Serves 2

Mushroom Salad

This salad can be prepared with any type of mushroom. Portobello mushrooms will add a good meaty side to the taste, and they will also absorb the marinade, making them extremely flavorful. Wild mushrooms are another variety that will add a pleasant, yet distinct taste to your salad. Any fresh green may be used — arugula and baby spinach are two wonderful options.

- 2 tablespoons plus ¼ cup shallots, finely chopped, divided
- 3 tablespoons rice vinegar
- 11 tablespoons olive oil, divided
- 2 pounds Portobello mushrooms, sliced
- 1 teaspoon fresh thyme
- Freshly ground black pepper, to taste
- 6 ounces fresh greens

In a small bowl, combine the 2 tablespoons shallots and vinegar. Beat the mixture together and set aside for 5 minutes to permit the shallots to absorb the vinegar. Once they have absorbed the vinegar, mix in 7 tablespoons of olive oil and set aside.

In a large skillet over a medium-high heat, add the remaining oil. Add in the mushrooms and sprinkle with the thyme and some pepper. Depending on what type of mushrooms you use, the cooking time will vary. Add the ¼ cup shallots in with the mushrooms and continue cooking until the shallots are soft. Season with freshly ground black pepper.

Fill a large plate or bowl with the fresh greens. Place the mushrooms from the skillet on top of the greens and top with the vinaigrette.

Serves 4

Walnut and Beet Salad

Beets are a valuable root vegetable, low in saturated fat and cholesterol and a good source of dietary fiber and vitamin C. However, most people are not familiar enough with beets to use them regularly. This salad offers a quick and tasty way to incorporate beets into your diet.

- 4 medium-sized red beets, stems and ends removed
- ⅓ cup walnuts, chopped
- 2 tablespoons balsamic vinegar
- 2 tablespoons olive oil
- Freshly ground black pepper, to taste

Preheat oven to 400 degrees F. Wrap each beet in foil and place on a baking sheet. Roast in the oven for just about an hour.

Remove beets from the oven and allow to cool. Once cool enough to handle, remove them from the foil. While still warm, remove the skin of the beets. Plastic gloves are suggested so you do not stain your hands.

Slice beets into large chunks. Place in a medium bowl and mix in the remaining ingredients. Season with freshly ground black pepper. Allow beets to saturate in the dressing prior to serving.

Serves 4

Hot Chicken and Zucchini Salad

This is a hot salad featuring the unique combination of chicken and zucchini that is simple to prepare. Top with fresh almonds to complement the lemon and garlic mayonnaise.

- 2 tablespoons plus ¼ cup shallots, finely chopped, divided
- 3 tablespoons rice vinegar
- 2 pounds chicken breasts, cut into cubes
- 3 tablespoons coconut oil
- 1 large onion, chopped
- 5 small zucchinis, cut into cubes
- 1 tablespoon dried oregano
- Freshly ground black pepper, to taste
- 7 tablespoons olive-oil mayonnaise
- Juice of 2 lemons
- 2 cloves garlic, minced very finely
- 1 head romaine lettuce, washed and shredded
- Sliced almonds, optional

Add the chicken cubes and coconut oil in a large pan over a medium-high heat until thoroughly cooked. Set aside.

Add the onion in the same pan and cook until soft, approximately 5 minutes.

Put in the zucchini cubes and oregano, and season with pepper. Cook until the zucchini cubes are soft.

Mix the mayonnaise, lemon juice, and garlic into a small bowl.

Add the cooked chicken, onion, and zucchini to the mayonnaise and stir well.

Add romaine lettuce, mix well, and serve in bowls. This hot salad is delicious topped with some almonds.

Serves 4

Salmon Salad

Heart-healthy salmon provides a hefty helping of omega-3 fatty acids for good brain and eye health. Use leftover grilled salmon in this tasty lunch salad.

- 1 cup cooked, flaked salmon
- ½ cup green onions, chopped
- ½ cup macadamia nuts, chopped
- ½ cup dried cranberries
- 4 cups mixed baby greens
- Freshly ground black pepper, to taste
- 2 tablespoons tahini paste
- 2 tablespoons sesame oil
- 2 tablespoons olive oil
- 1 teaspoon garlic, minced
- ½ teaspoon thyme

Combine the salmon, onions, nuts, cranberries, and baby greens in a large salad bowl. Season with freshly ground black pepper.

In a smaller bowl, whisk the remaining ingredients together to make an Asian-inspired dressing. Toss the dressing with the salad and serve immediately.

Serves 4

Tart Apple Coleslaw

This is a great side dish to bring to cookouts and is refreshingly sweet and tart from the addition of apples. Granny Smiths are the best choice for flavor and texture, but any apple will do in a pinch. If you use a sweet apple, you can omit the honey.

- ½ head green or purple cabbage, or a combination, grated
- 1 Granny Smith apple, grated
- 1 stalk celery, chopped
- 1 medium green pepper, diced
- ¼ cup olive oil
- Juice of 1 lemon
- 2 tablespoons honey
- 1 teaspoon celery seed
- Freshly ground black pepper, to taste
- Sliced almonds, optional

Combine all the ingredients in a bowl and toss well to mix. Chill for an hour or more before serving.

Serves 4

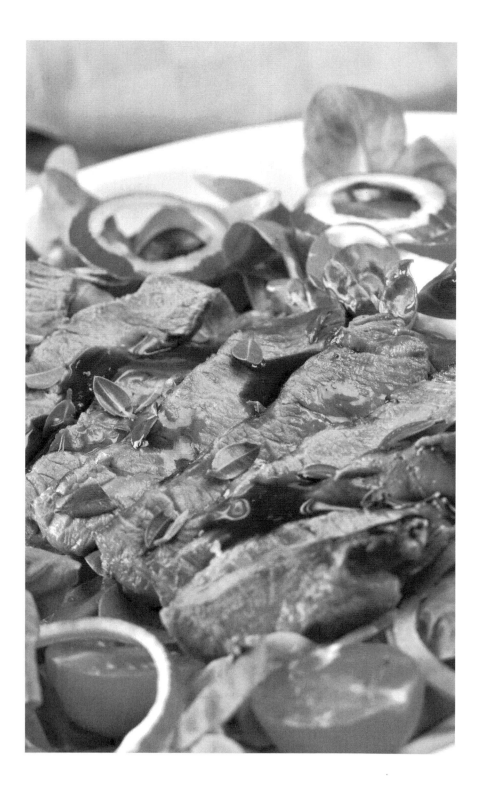

Robust Steak Salad

If you've limited your consumption of red meat in the past, rejoice! Red meat is allowed, and even encouraged on the Paleo diet. Seek out grass-fed beef from a reputable butcher. Grass-fed beef is higher in protein and lower in saturated fats than conventionally grown beef.

- 1 cup grass-fed steak, grilled and cut in thin slices
- ½ cup red onion, sliced in rings
- ½ cup cherry or grape tomatoes
- 4 cups baby greens
- Freshly ground black pepper, to taste
- ¼ cup red wine vinegar
- ½ teaspoon thyme
- 1 teaspoon dry mustard
- 1 teaspoon garlic, minced
- ½ cup olive oil

Combine the steak and vegetables in a salad bowl. Season with freshly ground black pepper.

Whisk the vinegar, spices, and garlic together in a smaller bowl. Add the olive oil in a slow drizzle, whisking until it becomes thick. Toss the dressing with the salad and serve immediately.

Serves 4

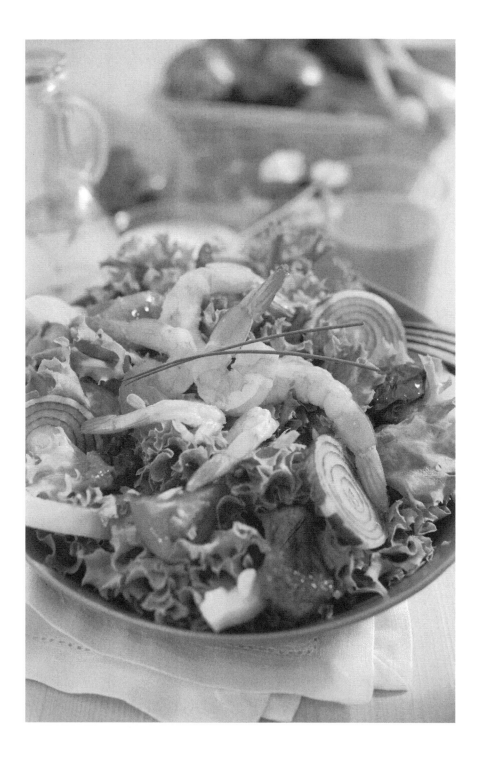

Savory Shrimp Salad

Shrimp, with its gently curving shape and delicate pink color, looks beautiful in salads and main dishes. It also pairs beautifully with bacon and avocado. Shrimp comes frozen in large bags labeled by the number of shrimp in each bag. The lower the number, the larger the shrimp. For this recipe, look for shrimp that has already been deveined and shelled.

- 1 cup shrimp, grilled or steamed
- 1 cup avocado, cubed
- ½ cup red onion, diced
- 2 strips of uncured, nitrate-free bacon, cooked and crumbled
- 4 cups baby greens
- ¼ cup fresh orange juice
- 1 teaspoon honey
- 1 teaspoon garlic, minced
- 1 teaspoon ginger powder
- Freshly ground black pepper, to taste
- ½ cup grapeseed oil

Combine the shrimp, avocado, red onions, bacon, and baby greens in a salad bowl.

In a smaller bowl, whisk the orange juice, honey, garlic, ginger powder, and black pepper. Slowly add the oil, whisking vigorously until it emulsifies.

Toss the dressing with the salad and serve immediately.

Serves 4

Classic Vinaigrette

This vinaigrette is a great basic dressing for almost any salad. The easiest way to prepare it is to put all ingredients in a jar and shake. Store in the jar and then you can shake again when you're ready to use more.

- ½ cup olive oil
- 3 tablespoons red wine vinegar
- 1 teaspoon Dijon mustard
- 1 garlic clove, minced
- 1 teaspoon honey
- Freshly ground black pepper, to taste

Put all ingredients in a jar, close the lid and shake until emulsified. Alternately, you can put everything in a blender and blend. Use to dress any salad right before serving and store the remaining dressing in the refrigerator for up to 3 days.

Makes ½ cup

Honey-Lime Vinaigrette

This is a great dressing for any southwestern-style salad. It pairs beautifully with tomatoes and avocado, and is even delicious on melon or peaches. Store extra in the refrigerator.

- ½ cup olive oil
- Juice of 1 lime
- 1 teaspoon honey
- ¼ teaspoon ground cumin
- Pinch chili powder
- Freshly ground black pepper, to taste

Put all ingredients in a jar or container with a lid and shake until combined. Use to dress salad right before serving.

Makes ½ cup

Orange Balsamic Vinaigrette

This sweet and tangy dressing gets its citrusy flavor from the addition of freshly squeezed orange juice and zest. The addition of mustard adds a little zip but also helps keep it from separating. This vinaigrette pairs beautifully over a spinach salad with fresh berries and red onions.

- ½ cup olive oil
- 2 tablespoons balsamic vinaigrette
- Juice and zest of one large orange
- 1 clove garlic, minced
- 1 teaspoon Dijon mustard
- Freshly ground black pepper, to taste

Put all ingredients in a jar or closed container and shake vigorously until emulsified. Use to dress salad right before serving and store any remaining dressing in the refrigerator for up to 3 days.

Makes ½ cup

Lemon Vinaigrette

This light and lemony dressing makes an excellent choice for a simple green salad without too many flavors and textures. It works beautifully on salads that have a grilled protein such as chicken or salmon as well, and you can easily customize it by adding herbs of your choice.

- ½ cup olive oil
- Juice of 1 lemon
- 1 teaspoon Dijon mustard
- 1 small clove garlic, minced
- Freshly ground black pepper, to taste

Put all ingredients in a jar or other container with a lid and shake until emulsified. Use to dress salad immediately before serving and refrigerate any remaining dressing for up to 3 days.

Makes ½ cup

Caesar Dressing

While you can't have croutons with a Paleo Caesar salad, if the dressing is flavorful enough, you don't really need them. This version fits the bill, and it's much healthier than most bottled dressings. This is delicious over a seared or grilled salmon fillet and some fresh and crisp romaine lettuce.

- ½ cup olive oil
- 2 tablespoons olive-oil mayonnaise
- 4 garlic cloves, minced
- Juice of 1 lemon
- 1 tablespoon Dijon mustard
- 1 tablespoon Worcestershire sauce
- 3 to 4 anchovy fillets if desired, minced
- Freshly ground black pepper, to taste

Combine all ingredients in a blender or food processor and blend until smooth and creamy. Toss romaine lettuce with the dressing, top with desired protein or vegetables, and serve.

Makes ½ cup

8

MAIN DISHES

Classic Diner Steak and Eggs

Two keystones of the Paleo diet, steak and eggs, make a classic combination that has been served for ages. This is a simple recipe that can be enjoyed in the morning for breakfast or in the evening for a quick dinner. The eggs can be prepared however you like, although traditional steak and eggs are prepared with sunny-side-up eggs.

- 2 tablespoons olive or coconut oil
- 1 grass-fed steak fillet of your choice
- Freshly ground black pepper, to taste
- 2 large eggs
- Paprika to taste

Heat a pan over a medium-high heat, and heat 1 tablespoon of the oil. Lightly season steak with freshly ground black pepper.

Cook the steak to your favorite temperature. Approximately 3 minutes on each side will usually give you a medium-rare steak.

Take out the steak, set aside, and lower the temperature to medium-low. Add the remaining oil.

Crack open the eggs in the hot pan, cover and cook them however you would like them prepared. Season with freshly ground black pepper and paprika. Serve with the steak immediately.

Serves 1

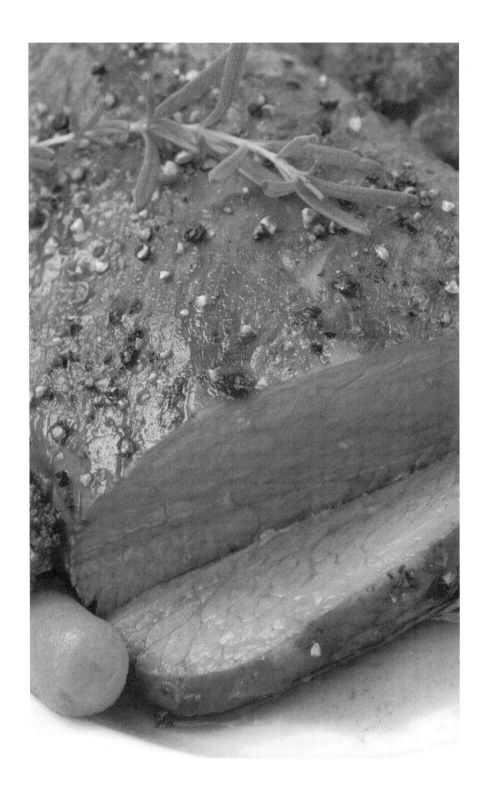

Beef Rib Roast with a Green Peppercorn Sauce

The next time you are in charge of cooking for guests, a prime beef rib roast is a delicious, juicy dish that will have them raving about the meal for years to come. This cooking method will create an amazing juice that is then used to create an unforgettable peppercorn sauce.

- 1 (6-pound) grass-fed beef rib roast
- 1 medium onion, chopped
- 3 garlic cloves, minced
- 1 medium carrot, sliced
- Pinch dried thyme
- 2 tablespoons olive or coconut oil plus additional as needed
- Freshly ground black pepper, to taste
- ½ cup organic red wine
- 1 cup beef stock
- 2 tablespoons green peppercorns

Preheat oven to 400 degrees F.

Trim some of the excess fat off the rib points and the roast itself. This fat will be used to help create the sauce.

Put the trimmed fat into a roasting pan and add the onion, garlic, carrot, and thyme.

Add a generous amount of olive or coconut oil. Place the pan in the oven and roast for approximately 20 minutes, or until golden.

Remove the pan from the oven, put the roast on top of the vegetables and fat parts, and season with pepper and some more thyme. Add more oil.

Place the pan with the roast back into the oven and roast for 45 minutes.

Lower the oven temperature to 350 degrees F and cook for another 45 minutes for a medium-rare roast.

Take the pan out of the oven and remove the roast. Set the roast aside, freely covered with a piece of parchment or aluminum foil, for approximately 15 minutes.

Place the roasting pan on the stovetop and deglaze it with red wine. Be sure to scrape the pan considerably with a wooden spoon. Boil and reduce the liquid to one-third. Add beef stock and boil for another 5 minutes.

Add the green peppercorns and squash them with a fork. Season with freshly ground black pepper.

Serve immediately with slices of rib roast.

Serves 8 to 10

Portobello Burgers

Pretty much anything goes when you are topping these burgers. Make sure to use a ground beef that is lean, but not too lean. You want a little bit of fat in the meat to add more flavor. Using the portobello mushrooms as the bun offers a nice alternative to bread, as well as a unique taste. Add your favorite vegetables, just as you would with any burger. Avocados add a nice taste as well.

- 3 pounds grass-fed ground beef
- 3 large eggs
- 2 cloves garlic, minced

- Freshly ground black pepper, to taste
- 8 to 12 large portobello mushrooms
- 2 tablespoons olive oil

Place ground beef in a bowl and mix with the eggs. Add in the garlic and season lightly with pepper. Form 6 to 8 patties that are smaller than the mushroom caps.

Put on a preheated grill and cook each side for about 5 to 7 minutes. Rinse mushrooms and pat dry. Remove the mushroom stems.

Coat the caps in olive oil and then season with pepper. Do not let the oil penetrate for long to keep the mushrooms from getting soggy.

Place on preheated grill and cook on each side for about 5 to 7 minutes. Add hamburger patty and top as desired.

Serves 4 to 6

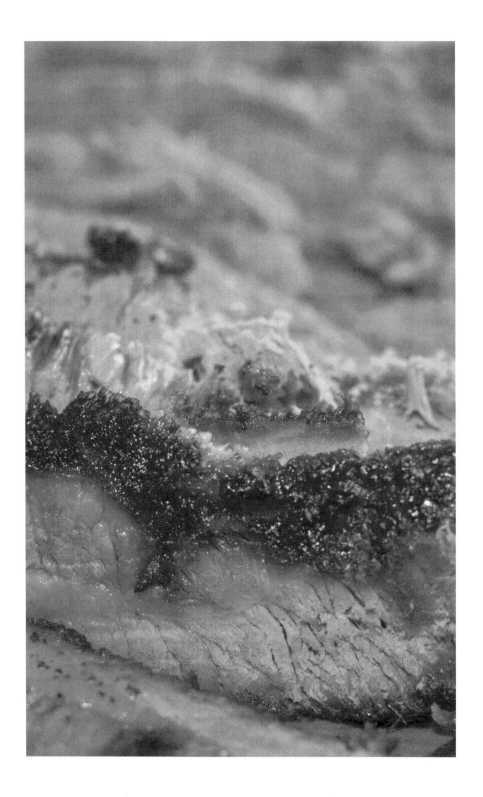

Tangy Beef Brisket

Beef brisket comes from the chest of the cow, and is tough and stringy. However, it's reasonably priced and has a lot of flavor. The secret is long, slow cooking. The acid in the tomato paste helps to tenderize this beef brisket, while the molasses gives it some sweetness.

- 1 (6-ounce) can tomato paste
- 2 tablespoons molasses
- 2 tablespoons cider vinegar
- 1 teaspoon dry mustard
- 1 teaspoon garlic, minced
- 2 tablespoons olive oil
- 2 pounds grass-fed beef brisket
- ½ cup onion, chopped
- Freshly ground black pepper, to taste

Mix the tomato paste, molasses, vinegar, mustard, and garlic in a bowl.

Heat the oil in a large skillet over medium heat. Add the beef brisket and brown it on all sides, about 10 minutes. Add the onions and cook until tender.

Transfer the brisket and onions to a slow cooker. Spoon the tomato mixture over the brisket. Season with freshly ground black pepper. Cook on low, 6 to 8 hours, until tender.

Serves 6

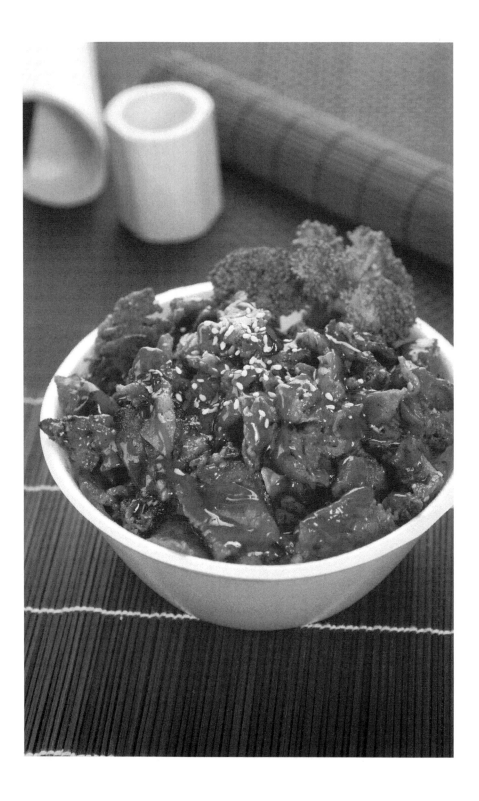

Slow Cooker Teriyaki Beef

The sugars in the honey become caramelized as this beef cooks, resulting in a sweet, tender, and highly flavorful meat. Serve it with stir-fried vegetables for a quick meal after work.

- 1 pound grass-fed flank steak or top sirloin, sliced thinly
- ¼ cup coconut aminos
- 1 tablespoon honey
- ½ teaspoon dried ginger
- 1 tablespoon tapioca
- Freshly ground black pepper, to taste
- 1 green onion, chopped

Place the steak in the slow cooker and turn on low.

Mix the aminos, honey, ginger, and tapioca in a bowl. Season with freshly ground black pepper. Pour this mixture over the steak and cover. Cook for 5 to 7 hours, or until very tender. Top with the green onions and serve.

Serves 4

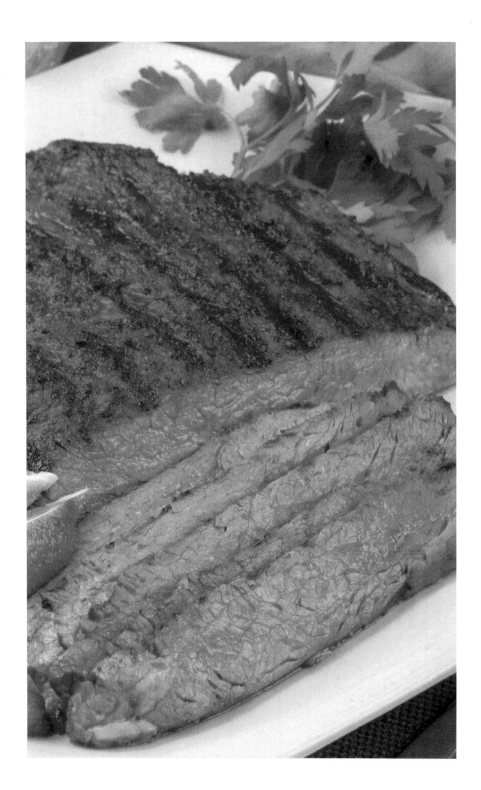

Roasted Citrus Flank Steak

Flank steak can be mouthwateringly delicious when done well, and this recipe does just that. The citrus marinade tenderizes an otherwise tough cut of meat, turning it into a succulent cut that pairs beautifully with simple grilled or steamed vegetables.

- Juice of 1 orange
- Juice of 3 limes
- 2 cloves garlic, minced
- 1 tablespoon Dijon mustard
- 1 tablespoon raspberry vinegar
- 2 pounds grass-fed flank steak
- Freshly ground black pepper, to taste

Combine the orange juice, lime juice, garlic, mustard, and vinegar in a gallon-size freezer bag. Add the flank steak and toss to coat evenly. Chill in the refrigerator for 1 hour.

Preheat oven to 400 degrees F. Lay the steak on a baking sheet or casserole dish and roast for 10 to 12 minutes. Remove from oven and allow to rest for 10 minutes before slicing and serving.

Serves 4

Zesty Meatloaf

Traditional meatloaf recipes call for breadcrumbs or crackers to bind the meat. This delicious alternative uses potato starch instead.

- 2 strips uncured, nitrate-free bacon, diced
- ½ cup onion, diced
- ½ cup red bell pepper, diced
- 1 pound grass-fed ground beef
- 1 large egg

- 2 tablespoons potato starch
- Freshly ground black pepper, to taste
- ½ cup ketchup
- 1 teaspoon dry mustard
- 1 tablespoon maple syrup

Preheat oven to 375 degrees F. Heat a skillet over medium heat. Add the bacon and cook for 4 to 5 minutes, or until brown and crisp. Transfer to a plate with a slotted spoon. Cook the diced onion and bell pepper in the bacon drippings until tender.

Combine the ground beef, egg, and potato starch in a medium bowl. Add the bacon, onions, and bell pepper, and stir gently to mix. Season with freshly ground black pepper. Pour the mixture into a loaf pan.

In another bowl, stir the ketchup, mustard, and maple syrup together. Pour this mixture over the meatloaf. Bake for 40 minutes, or until cooked through and brown on top.

Serves 4

Grilled Lamb Chops

If you're looking for something different to throw on the grill on a hot summer's night, why not try lamb chops? They're a great alternative to the usual chicken breasts or steaks. This version, with a simple garlic and lemon marinade, is easy to make and super delicious.

- ¼ cup olive oil
- 2 tablespoons lemon juice
- 3 cloves garlic, minced
- 1 small shallot, minced
- 1 teaspoon dried oregano
- Freshly ground black pepper, to taste
- 6 lamb chops

In a small bowl, combine the olive oil, lemon juice, garlic, shallot, and oregano. Season with freshly ground black pepper. Stir to combine well.

Put the lamb chops and the marinade in a gallon-size freezer bag and shake. Chill for at least 1 hour, and up to 24.

When ready to cook, preheat grill to high heat. Grill the chops for about 5 minutes per side. Allow to rest for 10 minutes and serve.

Serves 2

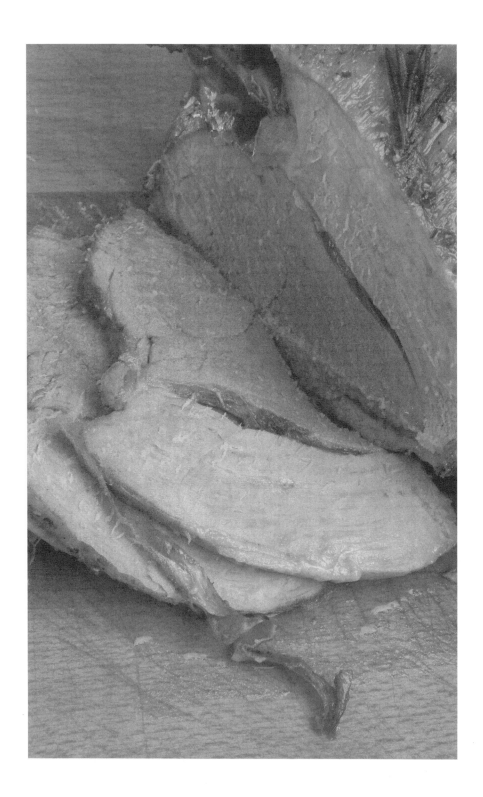

Leg of Lamb

Lamb is something typically served in the spring around the Easter holiday, but it's actually a meal that doesn't have to wait for a holiday celebration to be enjoyed. With only a few ingredients, you can enjoy this delicious dish anytime you want and still stick to your diet!

- 3 to 4 pounds boneless leg of lamb
- 1 garlic bulb, separated and peeled
- 2 tablespoons fresh thyme, chopped
- Freshly ground black pepper, to taste

Preheat oven to 325 degrees F. After peeling garlic cloves, push them into lamb leg all over. Rub the thyme all over the lamb leg and lightly season with pepper.

Roast for about 25 minutes per pound for medium-rare, or longer if desired. Allow to rest for 10 to 15 minutes before serving.

Serves 6 to 8

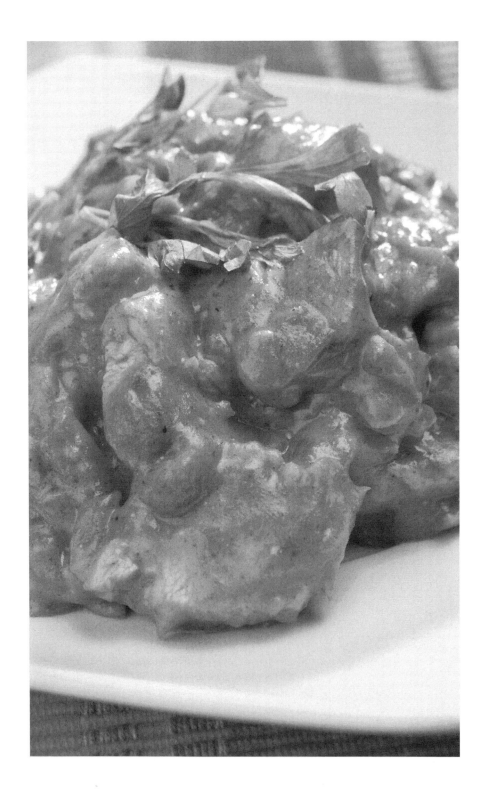

Green Chicken Masala

This recipe may have quite a few ingredients, but it is simple and quick, taking no more than 30 minutes to prepare. Similar to the traditional tikka masala, the combination of Indian spices gives a nice and spicy taste to this dish. You may substitute chicken thighs with pork or beef for equally great results.

- 1 onion, finely chopped
- 3 tablespoons olive or coconut oil
- 2 pounds skinless, boneless chicken thighs, cut into 1-inch pieces
- 1½ teaspoons turmeric
- ¼ cup lemon juice
- ½ cup water or chicken stock
- Small bunch fresh mint leaves
- 2 cups fresh cilantro leaves
- 1 jalapeño pepper, chopped coarsely
- 4 garlic cloves, minced
- ⅛ teaspoon ground cloves
- ½ teaspoon ground cardamom
- ½ teaspoon cinnamon
- 1 cup full-fat coconut milk
- Freshly ground black pepper, to taste

In a large skillet over medium heat, add the onion with the oil. Cook, stirring occasionally for approximately 5 minutes or until the onion starts to soften.

Add chicken thighs and the turmeric to the skillet and continue cooking, stirring occasionally for approximately another 7 minutes.

Place the lemon juice, water or stock, mint, cilantro, jalapeño, and garlic in a blender or food processor and blend until you obtain a smooth puree.

After the chicken has cooked for around 7 minutes, add the cloves, cardamom, and cinnamon. Cook for just about a minute.

Add in the coconut milk, season to taste with freshly ground black pepper and add the herb puree.

Bring it all to a nice simmer and let it continue for approximately 15 minutes, or until the chicken is well cooked and tender.

Serve immediately.

Serves 4

Thai Curry-Braised Chicken

You can control the heat of this dish by the amount of curry paste used. The coconut milk and ginger give it a sweet and spicy taste while creating a full-bodied flavor.

- 4 chicken legs and thighs
- 1 tablespoon olive oil
- Freshly ground black pepper, to taste
- ½ small onion, chopped
- 1 tablespoon fresh ginger, minced
- 2 cloves garlic, minced
- 1 tablespoon Thai red curry paste, to taste
- 1½ cups chicken broth
- 4 bok choy stalks
- 1 cup coconut milk
- Juice of 1 lime
- Fresh chopped cilantro for garnish

Preheat oven to 325 degrees F. Remove the skin from the chicken. Heat the oil in an ovenproof skillet with a lid over low heat. Season the chicken with pepper. Add chicken to the pan and sear on all sides. Take out the chicken and keep warm.

Stir in onions, ginger, and garlic and sauté until onions are soft, approximately 4 minutes. Stir in curry paste along with the broth. Season with freshly ground black pepper.

Place the chicken back in the pan and bring to a simmer. Transfer to oven and cook for 30 minutes.

Cut the bok choy stalks in half and put on a plate with a tiny amount of water, then cover with plastic wrap. Microwave on high for 2 minutes.

Remove pan from oven, remove chicken and reserve. Bring the liquid to a simmer and stir in the coconut milk. Add in lime juice and simmer for 2 minutes. Add the cilantro and return the chicken to the pan.

Place 2 bok choy halves onto each plate. Portion 1 drumstick and thigh on each plate. Spoon sauce over chicken and garnish with more cilantro, if desired.

Serves 4

Caveman Chicken Nuggets

Looking for a Paleo meal to entice your youngest cavemen? These tasty chicken nuggets are full of protein, but lack the sodium and preservatives found in commercial chicken nuggets. They're so good, in fact, you may have to fight your kids for them. Make a few extra and freeze them for easy lunch meals.

- 2 large egg whites
- ½ teaspoon garlic powder
- ½ teaspoon thyme
- ½ teaspoon rosemary
- 1 cup almond meal
- ½ cup pecans, finely chopped
- Freshly ground black pepper, to taste
- 1 pound boneless, skinless chicken breast, cut in 1½-inch cubes

Preheat oven to 375 degrees F.

Place the egg whites in a shallow dish. Mix the dry ingredients and spices in another shallow dish.

Lightly season the chicken pieces and dip the cubes in the egg whites and then the breading, coating them well. Place the chicken nuggets on a baking sheet and bake for 20 to 25 minutes. Serve immediately.

Serves 4

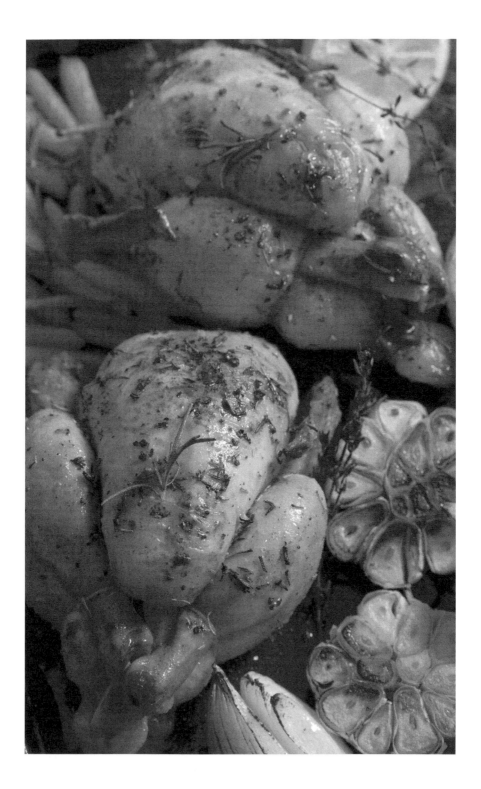

Lemon and Garlic Roasted Chicken

There is nothing much more elegant or delicious than a properly roasted chicken. While it can be intimidating the first time you do it, the truth is that it's much simpler than you think, and can be done for a regular weeknight meal. This lemon and garlic version is mouthwateringly succulent. Once you try it, it will surely be in your regular dinner rotation.

- 1 whole chicken
- 1 lemon
- 2 cloves garlic, minced
- 1 tablespoon fresh rosemary, chopped
- Freshly ground black pepper, to taste
- 2 tablespoons olive oil

Preheat oven to 350 degrees F.

Clean the chicken by removing the giblets and neck and rinsing the entire chicken. Dry thoroughly with paper towels. Put the chicken in a roasting pan, breast side up.

Zest the lemon. Combine the garlic, rosemary, lemon zest, black pepper, and olive oil in a small bowl and brush the mixture over the entire chicken, including inside the bird.

Slice the lemon and stuff the slices inside the cavity of the chicken.

Roast for 25 minutes per pound until the breast temperature reads 170 degrees F on an instant-read thermometer.

Allow chicken to rest for 10 minutes before carving and serving.

Serves 4

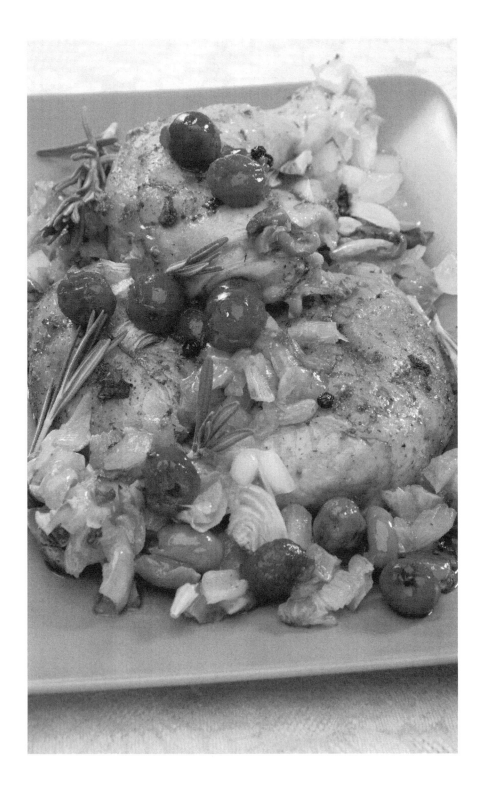

Fresh Cherry and Herbs Chicken

A variety of herbs give this chicken dish an amazing flavor. Lots of fresh cherries and almonds push it over the top. This chicken dish is savory, sweet, and crunchy all at the same time.

- 2 tablespoons olive oil, divided
- 2 shallots, thinly sliced
- 2 cups cherries, pitted and halved
- ⅛ cup red wine vinegar
- ¼ cup balsamic vinegar
- 2 teaspoons cinnamon
- 2 tablespoons dried tarragon
- 1 teaspoon ground ginger
- ½ teaspoon dried oregano
- ½ teaspoon dried thyme
- Freshly ground black pepper, to taste
- 1 pound chicken thighs
- 1 cup sliced almonds

Add 1 tablespoon olive oil to a large sauté pan over medium heat. Stirring occasionally, cook the shallots until translucent (3 to 4 minutes).

Add the cherries, vinegars, cinnamon, tarragon, ginger, oregano, thyme, and pepper. Turn heat down low and simmer for 10 minutes.

Meanwhile, heat another pan over medium-high heat with the remaining tablespoon of oil.

Add the chicken and cook until done (about 12 minutes), turning once.

Heat up a small sauté pan and add the almonds.

Toast the almonds, constantly shaking the pan, until they are lightly toasted and you can smell them.

Divide the chicken among dinner plates.

Pour the sauce over the chicken and garnish with the sliced almonds.

Serves 4 to 5

Venison Medallions with Quick Mustard Sauce

If you haven't been around hunters or hunted your own meat, you may have never tried venison, which is deer meat. While it does taste similar to beef in dishes like tacos, it does have a unique flavor that stands out in this dish. If you know a hunter and can get fresh venison, do so; otherwise, meat from a butcher will do.

- 3 tablespoons Dijon mustard, divided
- 1 to 2 pounds venison tenderloin, cut into medallions ½-inch thick
- 1 tablespoon olive or coconut oil, divided
- 1 shallot, minced
- Freshly ground black pepper, to taste
- 1½ cups beef stock

Rub 1 tablespoon of the mustard into the medallions. Heat a large skillet over medium-high heat and add 1 tablespoon of oil. When the pan is very hot, add the venison to the pan, cooking in batches if necessary. Sear for 4 minutes per side and remove from the pan.

Add the remaining oil and shallots to the same pan and reduce the heat, scraping up any browned bits. Season with freshly ground black pepper.

Add the stock and remaining mustard and whisk to create a smooth sauce.

To serve, drizzle the sauce over the venison medallions.

Serves 4

Nectarine and Onion Pork Chops

Apples are frequently coupled with pork, but other fruits can do a noble job, too, as the nectarines do in this recipe. Try out a variation of different fruits with the recipe, such as grapes or berries.

- 3 nectarines, pitted and chopped
- 1 large onion, cut into quarters
- 2 tablespoons olive or coconut oil
- Freshly ground black pepper, to taste
- 6 bone-in pork chops
- Juice of 1 lemon
- 1 tablespoon Dijon mustard
- 1 small bunch fresh mint, chopped

Combine the nectarine and onion in a bowl with the oil and season the mixture to taste with freshly ground black pepper.

Heat a large skillet over medium heat, put in the nectarine and onion mixture and cook, stirring frequently or until the nectarine pieces have softened, approximately 8 minutes.

Set aside to cool. Wipe the skillet clean to cook the pork chops.

Rub additional oil on the pork chops on both sides and season them to taste with pepper. Reheat skillet to a medium heat. Add the chops to the hot skillet and cook for about 3 minutes per side or until well cooked.

When the pork chops are cooking, cut the cooked nectarine and onion quarters into ¼-inch thick slices. Place the slices back into the bowl with their juices.

Mix the lemon juice, mustard, and chopped mint into the nectarine and onion mixture.

Serve the cooked pork chops topped with the nectarine mixture.

Serves 6

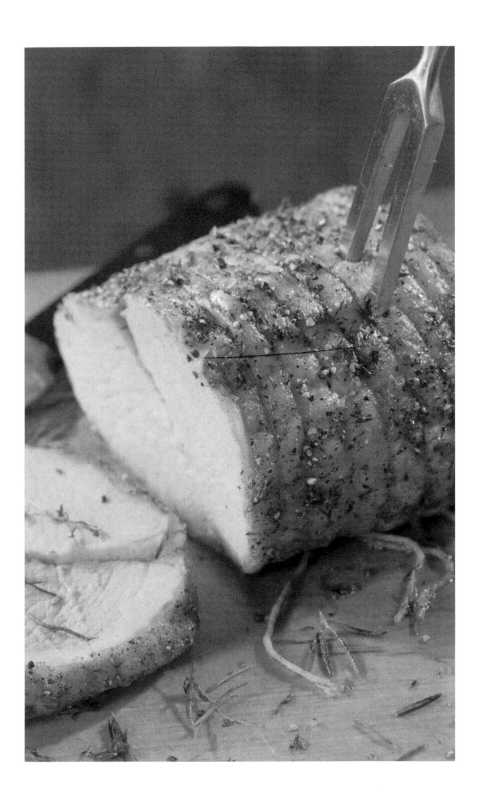

Slow Roasted Pork Roast

One of the best things about the Paleo diet is that it includes a lot of your favorite comfort foods. (Okay, not all of them, but who needs mac 'n' cheese when you can eat this pork roast?) Serve this with a green salad drizzled with olive oil for a complete and satisfying meal you'll make again and again.

- 2 tablespoons olive oil
- 4-pound pork roast
- 1 small onion, sliced
- 2 garlic cloves, smashed
- 2 sweet potatoes, peeled and diced
- 1 cup tomatoes, diced
- 1 bay leaf
- 2 cups chicken or beef stock
- Freshly ground black pepper, to taste

Preheat oven to 325 degrees F. In a large Dutch oven, add the oil and pork roast. Sear until deeply browned on all sides. Remove and set aside.

Add onions and garlic to the pot and cook until softened. Add sweet potatoes, tomatoes, bay leaf, and stock. Bring to a boil and reduce heat to a simmer. Season with freshly ground black pepper.

Simmer for 2 hours and then turn oven down to 250 degrees F and continue cooking until roast is tender, about 2 to 3 more hours. Serve immediately.

Serves 4 to 6

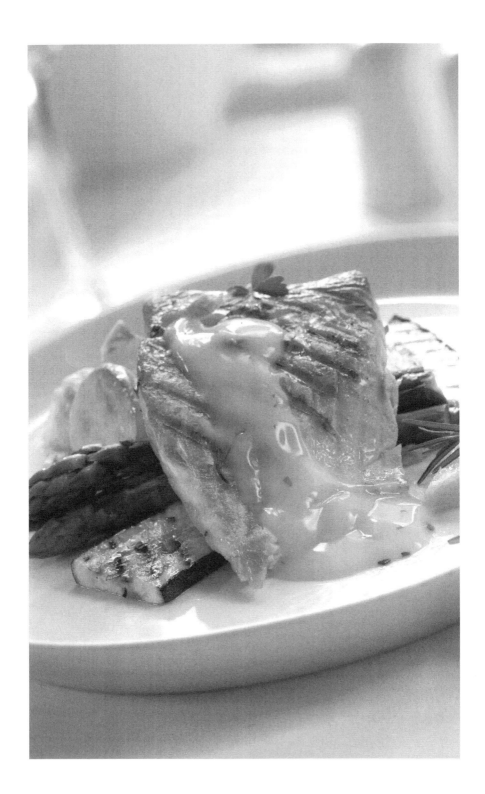

Slow Roasted Salmon with Hollandaise

Hollandaise sauce needs to be served warm, and should be made right before serving it—but it goes together in a snap to give this salmon a creamy finish.

- 14 tablespoons olive or coconut oil
- 4 salmon fillets
- 4 large, cage free, organic egg yolks
- Juice of 1 lemon
- ¼ teaspoon cayenne pepper
- Freshly ground black pepper, to taste

Melt 2 tablespoons of the olive or coconut oil in a large frying pan, reserving the remaining or coconut oil. Place the salmon in the hot frying pan and cook it for 8-12 minutes, turning halfway through the cooking time.

Melt the remaining olive or coconut oil in the microwave. Blend the egg yolks, lemon juice and peppers in a blender. Slowly add the melted olive or coconut oil, a few drops at a time, and continue blending until the mixture emulsifies and becomes thick.

To serve, position the salmon over roasted asparagus or steamed bok choy. Drizzle the dish with the Hollandaise sauce.

Serves 4

Paleo Lasagna

If you find that you crave pasta on the Paleo diet, you'll be surprised to find that you do have some options. One of them is this delicious lasagna that will satisfy your craving for the comforting casserole. A mandolin will yield the best results as far as the zucchini slices go, but you can slice it with a sharp knife if necessary.

- 1 pound grass-fed ground beef
- 3 cloves garlic, minced
- 1 small onion, chopped
- 1 small green bell pepper, diced
- 6 ounces tomato paste
- 1 (15-ounce) can tomato sauce
- 1 tablespoon fresh parsley, chopped
- 2 tablespoons Italian seasoning
- Freshly ground black pepper, to taste
- 1 large zucchini, thinly sliced lengthwise
- 1 cup mushrooms, sliced

Preheat oven to 350 degrees F. In a large pot over medium heat, brown the beef while continuously stirring.

Add the garlic, onion, and bell pepper and continue cooking for about 5 more minutes.

Stir in the tomato paste and sauce, followed by the herbs. Season with freshly ground black pepper.

Bring to a boil and remove from heat.

In a 9 x 13-inch casserole dish, place a thin layer of the sauce. Layer the zucchini and mushrooms over the sauce and alternate layers until they reach the top or you run out of ingredients.

Cover with foil and bake for 25 to 30 minutes. Remove foil and bake for an additional 5 minutes. Allow to rest for 5 minutes before serving.

Serves 8

Paleo Spaghetti and Meat Sauce

If you haven't tried spaghetti squash, you're in for a treat. The squash has a sweet, mellow flavor and forms spaghetti-like strands when cooked. Serve it with this hearty, slow-cooker meat sauce for a filling lunch or dinner.

- 1 pound grass-fed ground beef
- ½ cup onion, chopped
- ½ cup celery, chopped
- ½ cup carrots, chopped
- 2 teaspoons garlic, minced
- 3 (14-ounce) cans tomato puree
- 1 (8-ounce) can tomato paste
- ½ cup organic red wine
- 1 teaspoon thyme
- 1 teaspoon marjoram
- 1 spaghetti squash
- Freshly ground black pepper, to taste

Brown the ground beef in a large skillet. Add the vegetables and cook them until they are tender. Transfer the ground beef and vegetables to a slow cooker, and add the remaining ingredients except the spaghetti squash.

Preheat oven to 350 degrees F. Cut the squash in half and remove the seeds. Place the squash in a baking pan, cut side down. Fill the pan with 2 inches of hot water. Cover with aluminum foil and bake for 40 minutes, or until tender. Scoop the squash out and place it in a serving dish. Serve with the meat sauce.

Serves 6

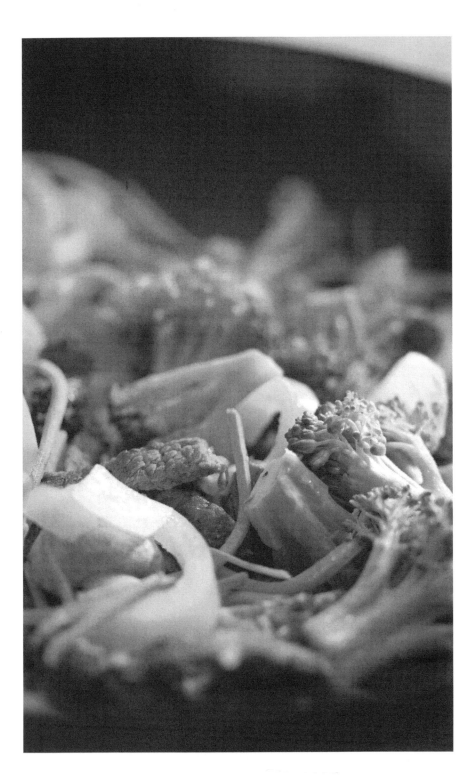

Beef Stir-Fry

You'll have to eat this stir-fry without rice if you're trying to stick to the diet, but with the flavor from high-quality beef, it's unlikely you'll miss it. As with all cooking, you want to buy the highest quality beef you can find, not only for flavor, but for health reasons as well.

- 1 pound grass-fed beef round, sliced into thin strips
- 2 tablespoons olive oil
- 1 garlic clove, minced
- 1 cup broccoli florets
- 1 cup carrots, sliced
- 1 cup snow pea pods
- ½ head cabbage, finely shredded
- 1 teaspoon apple cider vinegar
- Freshly ground black pepper, to taste
- Sesame seeds for garnish, if desired

Heat a large, non-stick skillet or wok over medium-high heat. Add sliced beef and cook until browned on all sides, almost cooked through. Remove from pan and set aside.

Add oil to pan, add garlic, followed by vegetables and vinegar. Stir-fry until crisp and tender. Season with freshly ground black pepper.

Add beef back to pan and finish cooking. Divide into bowls, top with sesame seeds, if desired, and serve immediately.

Serves 4

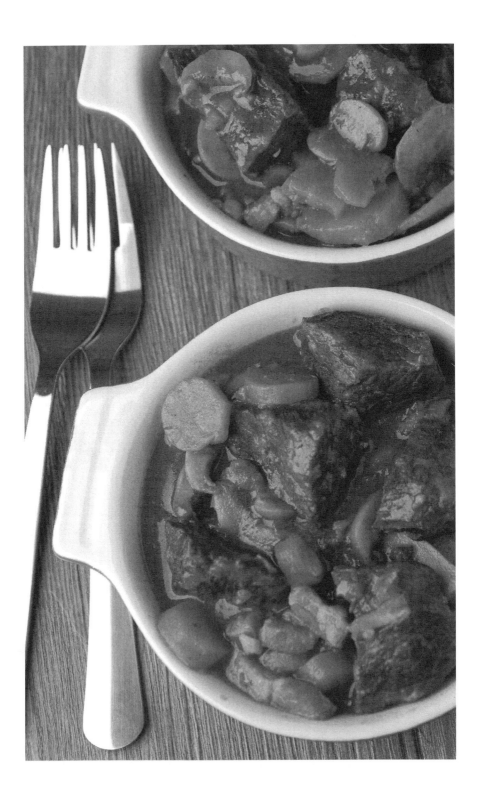

Beef Burgundy

Beef burgundy is traditionally served with mashed potatoes or noodles, but you won't miss them. This flavorful French stew is teeming with veggies and savory meat. Best of all, it cooks in the slow cooker, making it suitable for even a weeknight meal. Combine the ingredients the night before and refrigerate. In the morning, just turn the slow cooker on and dinner is made.

- 2 slices uncured, nitrate-free bacon
- ½ cup onion, chopped
- 1 teaspoon garlic, minced
- 1 pound grass-fed beef stew meat
- 5 carrots, peeled and diced
- 2 cups beef broth
- 1 cup organic red wine
- 3 tablespoons quick-cooking tapioca
- 3 tablespoons tomato paste
- ½ teaspoon thyme
- Freshly ground black pepper, to taste
- 2 tablespoons olive or coconut oil
- ½ cup mushrooms, chopped

Cook the bacon in a large skillet over medium heat. Crumble and transfer to the slow cooker. Add the onion and garlic to the bacon drippings and cook until tender. Brown the stew meat in the bacon drippings and transfer it to the slow cooker.

Add the carrots, broth, wine, tapioca, tomato paste, thyme, and pepper to the slow cooker. Cook on low for 6 to 8 hours.

Heat the oil in a small skillet and sauté the mushrooms for 5 to 7 minutes, or until tender. Stir the mushrooms into the stew and serve.

Serves 4

Pulled Pork with Homemade Barbecue Sauce

Pork roast is delicious cooked in the slow cooker. It becomes moist and savory. Commercial barbecue sauce is laden with high fructose corn syrup, sugar, and vinegar, but this homemade version is much healthier—and just as yummy.

- 2 tablespoons olive oil
- 2-pound boneless pork roast
- 1 teaspoon garlic, minced
- Freshly ground black pepper, to taste
- 1 (28-ounce) can tomato puree
- ½ cup onion, chopped
- ½ cup chicken broth

- ½ cup cider vinegar
- ¼ cup molasses
- 1 teaspoon dry mustard
- ¼ teaspoon ground cinnamon
- ¼ teaspoon ground allspice
- ¼ teaspoon ground cloves
- ¼ teaspoon ground ginger
- ¼ teaspoon ground red pepper flakes

Heat the olive oil in a skillet. Add the pork roast and brown slightly. Browning caramelizes the meat and improves its flavor. Place the pork roast in a slow cooker and add the garlic. Season with freshly ground black pepper. Cook on low for 3 to 4 hours, or until tender. Remove and shred.

Puree the tomatoes and onions in a food processor or blender. Add the pureed tomato and onions and remaining ingredients to the slow cooker, mixing well. Cook an additional 2 hours to meld the flavors.

Serves 4

Paleo Ratatouille

Ratatouille is the perfect vegetarian dinner for a warm, summer evening. Roast the season's bounty to bring out the flavors of the vegetables. Eggplant has a meaty texture and will fill you up without the addition of meat. Choose the freshest vegetables you can find—preferably from your own garden.

- 2 cups eggplant, cubed
- 1 red onion, peeled and slivered
- 3 carrots, peeled and sliced
- 1 cup zucchini rounds
- 1 large green bell pepper, sliced
- 1 large red bell pepper, sliced
- 1 cup summer squash rounds
- 2 fresh plum tomatoes, seeded and quartered
- Freshly ground black pepper, to taste
- 2 tablespoons olive oil
- 1 teaspoon garlic, minced
- 1 teaspoon thyme
- ½ teaspoon marjoram

Preheat oven to 425 degrees F. Spread the vegetables out on a large baking sheet. Season with freshly ground black pepper.

Mix the olive oil, garlic and herbs in a bowl. Drizzle over the vegetables and stir to coat them.

Roast for 15 to 20 minutes, until the vegetables are tender and glistening.

Serves 4

Winter Veggie Stew

This hearty stew is vegan, but it's also very filling. Many people are surprised to find that a lot of vegan dishes fit on the Paleo plan, and that it is quite possible to not eat meat and get a lot protein. Leafy greens, such as the kale and spinach in this dish, are loaded with fiber and protein, as well as vitamins and minerals that will keep your body going all day long.

- 2 tablespoons olive oil
- 1 small onion, minced
- 2 cloves garlic, minced
- 2 carrots, sliced
- 1 cup mushrooms, sliced
- 1 stalk celery, chopped
- 1 tablespoon Italian seasoning
- 4 cups packed baby spinach
- 1 large bunch Tuscan kale, chopped
- Freshly ground black pepper, to taste
- 6 cups vegetable broth
- 1 (15-ounce) can of chopped tomatoes

Heat the oil in a large soup pot or Dutch oven over medium heat. Add the onions, garlic, carrots, mushrooms, and celery and cook for 10 minutes until veggies are soft.

Add the Italian season, spinach, and kale and stir until everything is combined. Season with freshly ground black pepper.

Add the vegetable broth and tomatoes with juices. Bring to a boil. Reduce heat and simmer for 20 minutes until carrots are soft. Serve immediately.

Serves 4

9

SIDE DISHES AND SAUCES

Roasted Broccoli

If you only eat steamed broccoli, then this roasted variety will be a real treat. It doesn't take much more effort, but it takes on a whole new dimension thanks to a hot oven that caramelizes the tender green stems. Serve this alongside any meat or seafood for a delicious and healthy side you'll love.

- 1 pound broccoli florets, trimmed into bite-sized pieces
- 2 tablespoons olive oil
- Juice of 1 lemon
- Freshly ground black pepper, to taste

Preheat oven to 400 degrees F.

Lay broccoli on a parchment-lined sheet tray and drizzle with olive oil and lemon juice. Season with freshly ground black pepper.

Bake for 30 minutes, stirring halfway through, until the broccoli is slightly browned and crispy. Serve immediately.

Serves 4

Balsamic Roasted Onions

You may not think of onions as being a side dish, but once you've tried these sweet, delicate morsels, you'll quickly change your mind. Slice the onions with a mandolin to make sure the slices are all equal, ensuring that they'll cook evenly. Use these to top steaks and chops, or even to garnish soups or salads. Once you get creative, you'll find endless uses for them.

- 1 large red onion, sliced thinly
- 1 tablespoon olive oil
- Freshly ground black pepper, to taste
- 1 tablespoon balsamic vinegar
- ¼ teaspoon ground red pepper flakes

Preheat oven to 400 degrees F.

Lay the sliced onions in a baking dish in a single layer. Drizzle with olive oil. Season with freshly ground black pepper.

Roast for 30 minutes until onions start crisping and browning. Toss cooked onions with the balsamic vinegar and serve.

Serves 4

Crispy Lemon Green Beans

Lemon adds a touch of acidity that brings out the great flavor of fresh green beans. Roasting the beans in the oven makes them crispy and gives them an unexpected crunch you'll love.

- 1 pound of fresh green beans
- 2 tablespoons olive or coconut oil
- 2 teaspoons of dried rosemary
- 2 teaspoons of dried sage
- Freshly ground black pepper, to taste
- 1 lemon, thinly sliced, seeds removed

Preheat oven to 400 degrees F.

Add washed and trimmed green beans to a casserole dish. Pour oil over top of beans.

Sprinkle rosemary and sage, and mix ingredients until well coated. Season with freshly ground black pepper.

Place the lemon slices in an even layer over the green beans. Bake for 30 to 35 minutes until they are crispy.

Serves 4

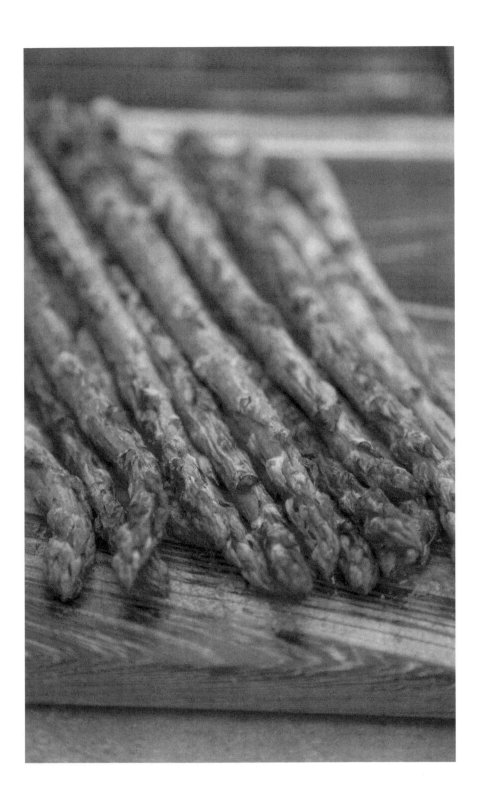

Simple Grilled Asparagus

Depending on the dish you are serving, sometimes you want a side dish with a lot of competing flavors and textures. Other times, though, you just want something that is good, but that won't outshine your main course. That's the case with this simple grilled asparagus recipe. It's one vegetable, and it's amazing when grilled, but when you serve it alongside a tender steak, it complements rather than takes center stage. It's also easy to make, and will make any meal feel like a special occasion.

- 1 pound asparagus stalks, tough ends trimmed
- 1 tablespoon olive oil
- Freshly ground black pepper, to taste
- Lemon juice, for seasoning

Preheat a gas or charcoal grill to medium-high heat. Toss the asparagus with olive oil and season with freshly ground black pepper and lemon juice.

Lay the asparagus on the grill grates diagonally so that they don't fall through. Cook for 5 to 6 minutes, turning consistently, until they are tender.

Remove from grill and serve immediately.

Serves 4

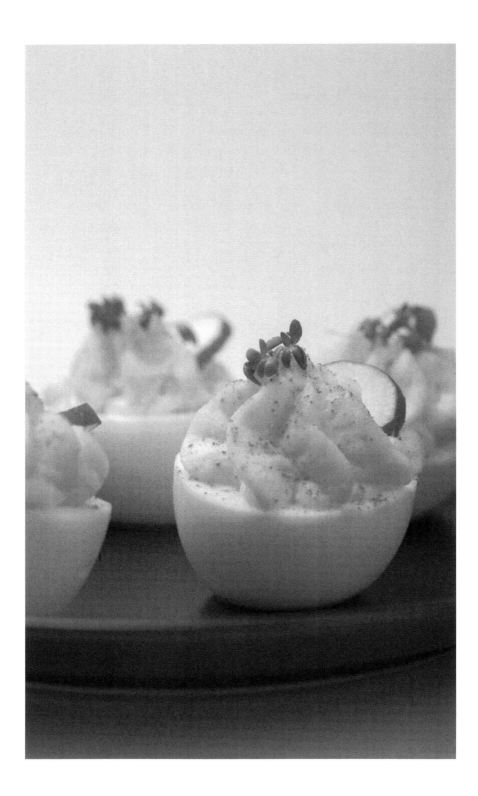

Deviled Eggs with Bacon Bits

Deviled eggs are a classic appetizer, but can also be used as a nice side dish for lighter lunches and dinners. They are easy to prepare and universally enjoyed, especially with this recipe that adds bacon bits for a nice, unexpected flavor.

- 6 slices uncured, nitrate-free bacon
- 12 large eggs
- cup olive-oil mayonnaise
- 1 tablespoon mustard
- 1 tablespoon ground cumin
- Freshly ground black pepper, to taste
- Paprika for garnish

Cook bacon in a pan over medium heat until crispy. Let cool and crumble into small bits.

Place eggs in a pot filled with cold water. Bring to a boil for 12 minutes. Remove from the heat, drain, and add cold water immediately to the eggs.

Once the eggs are cool enough to handle, peel and cut in half.

Scoop out the yolks and mash in a bowl with mayonnaise, mustard, cumin, bacon bits, and pepper.

Fill in the cavity of the egg white halves with the yolk, mayonnaise, and bacon filling.

Garnish with paprika or any of your favorite fresh herbs.

Makes 2 dozen

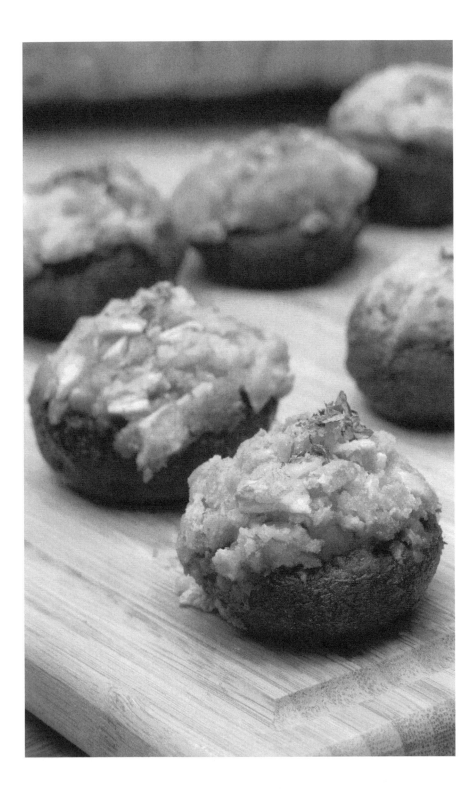

Crab-Stuffed Mushrooms

Mushrooms can often be forgotten on a Paleo diet, but they are certainly a healthy and tasty addition to any recipe. Mushrooms are often stuffed with cheeses, but these crab-stuffed ones are just as delectable. Simple white button mushrooms are perfect here, but feel free to use any mushroom you have handy that are big enough to stuff.

- 20 button mushrooms, stems and gills removed
- 2 cups crabmeat, cooked and finely chopped
- 3 tablespoons chives, minced
- 3 cloves garlic, minced
- ¼ teaspoon dried oregano
- ¼ teaspoon dried thyme
- ¼ teaspoon mustard
- Freshly ground black pepper, to taste

Preheat oven to 350 degrees F.

Mix all the ingredients except mushrooms together in a bowl. Spoon a generous portion into each mushroom and bake on a baking sheet for about 15 minutes.

Let cool slightly, but serve when still warm.

Serves 2 to 4

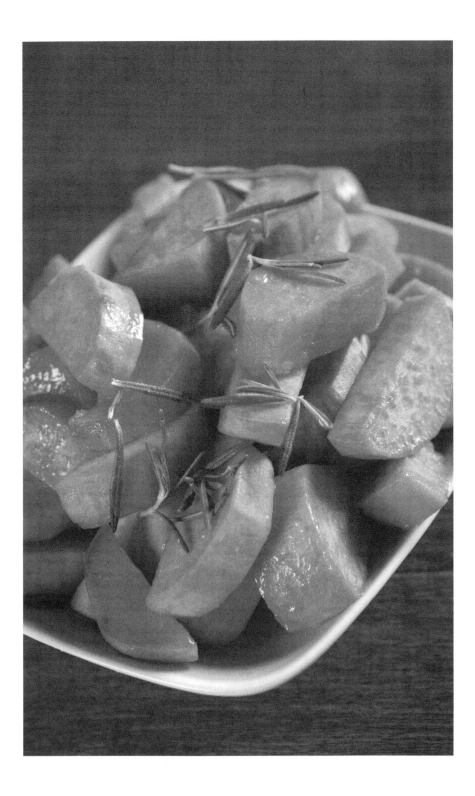

Roasted Sweet Potatoes with Rosemary

To make things a little unusual while keeping with the bulkier and orange autumn vegetables, this roasted, cubed, sweet potato dish with a touch of rosemary is perfect for any occasion. Rosemary features strong antioxidant assets, but feel free to use any woody herb such as thyme or sage in place of the rosemary.

- 2 large sweet potatoes, peeled and cut into 1-inch cubes
- 1 large sprig rosemary leaves
- 3 tablespoons olive or coconut oil
- 4 cloves garlic, crushed
- Freshly ground black pepper, to taste

Preheat oven to 425 degrees F.

Fill a pot with cold water, place in the sweet potato cubes, and bring to a rapid boil for 5 minutes. Quickly drain the potatoes in a colander and let steam and dry.

Using a mortar and pestle, grind the rosemary leaves.

Heat a roasting pan on the stove over medium-low heat, add the oil, rosemary, and sweet potato cubes and season with pepper. Stir until all ingredients are blended and hot.

Place the roasting pan in the oven and roast for approximately 20 to 25 minutes or until crispy and tender. Be sure to stir the potatoes occasionally for an even texture.

Serve warm.

Serves 2 to 4

Brussels Sprouts with Hazelnuts

This is a very simple way to roast Brussels sprouts, leaving them tender and full of flavor. Watch the hazelnuts carefully in the oven so they don't burn.

- 3 tablespoons olive or coconut oil
- 1 pound Brussels sprouts, trimmed and halved or quartered, depending on size
- ¼ cup hazelnuts, chopped
- Freshly ground black pepper, to taste

Preheat oven to 450 degrees F.

Toss the Brussels sprouts and hazelnuts with the oil and put onto a cookie sheet.

Sprinkle with pepper and place sheet into oven.

Bake for 15 minutes, occasionally turning the Brussels sprouts with a wooden spoon.

Serves 4

Kale with Walnuts and Cranberries

Kale is a good source of protein and vitamins. Cranberries and walnuts add excellent flavor to this side dish that goes great with beef or chicken. If you can find cranberries that have no added sugar, you should get those; otherwise, use dried tart cherries.

- 1 pound bunch of kale with tough stems removed, washed and torn into large pieces
- 2 tablespoons olive oil
- ½ medium red onion, finely chopped
- 3 cloves garlic, minced
- ½ cup walnuts, chopped
- ¼ cup dried cranberries, preferably with no added sugar
- Freshly ground black pepper, to taste

Bring a large of pot of water to a boil. Add the kale and cook until tender and bright green, about 4 or 5 minutes. Remove the kale and run under cold water to cool.

In a large sauté pan, add the oil over medium heat. Add the onion and sauté until soft.

Stir in the garlic and walnuts and cook until the nuts are golden, about 2 minutes. Mix the cranberries in, and then add the kale.

Toss gently with the onion/cranberry mixture. Season with pepper and serve warm.

Serves 2

Sweet Potato Mash with Pecans

Mashed sweet potatoes are very easy to prepare and do not require ingredients that you probably don't already have, which is always a plus. When eaten by themselves, sweet potatoes can be quite sweet. However, the green onions add a bite, and the pecans give a terrific nutty taste and add a nice, crunchy texture.

- 3 large sweet potatoes, peeled and cubed
- ½ cup olive or coconut oil
- Freshly ground black pepper, to taste
- 2 green onions, chopped
- ⅛ teaspoon ground cinnamon
- ¼ cup toasted pecans, chopped

Boil potatoes in large pot until soft enough to mash.

Strain the potatoes and put them back in the pot. Add the oil and mash until potatoes are smooth and silky. Season with freshly ground black pepper.

Add onions with the cinnamon and mix completely to ensure the cinnamon is dispersed consistently. Add the pecans.

Serve warm.

Serves 4

Paleo Barbecue Sauce

Most store-bought barbecue sauces are going to be loaded with sugar, even if they don't taste particularly sweet. This homemade version is spicy and complex—perfect for slow-cooked meats, grilled chicken, or anywhere else you would use barbecue sauce.

- 1 tablespoon olive or coconut oil
- 2 cloves garlic, minced
- 2 shallots, minced
- 1 teaspoon spicy brown mustard
- 1 teaspoon smoked paprika
- 1 teaspoon chili powder
- 1 teaspoon ground cumin
- 1 cup chicken broth
- Juice of 1 lime
- 1 (6-ounce) can tomato paste
- Freshly ground black pepper, to taste

In a medium saucepan, heat the oil over medium heat. Add the shallots and garlic. Cook until soft, about 3 minutes.

Add the mustard and spices and continue to cook, stirring for 1 more minute.

Add the broth, lime juice, and tomato paste and bring to a boil. Season with freshly ground black pepper.

Reduce to a simmer and cook for about 45 minutes. Allow to cool. For a smooth sauce, puree in a blender or food processor.

Makes 2 cups

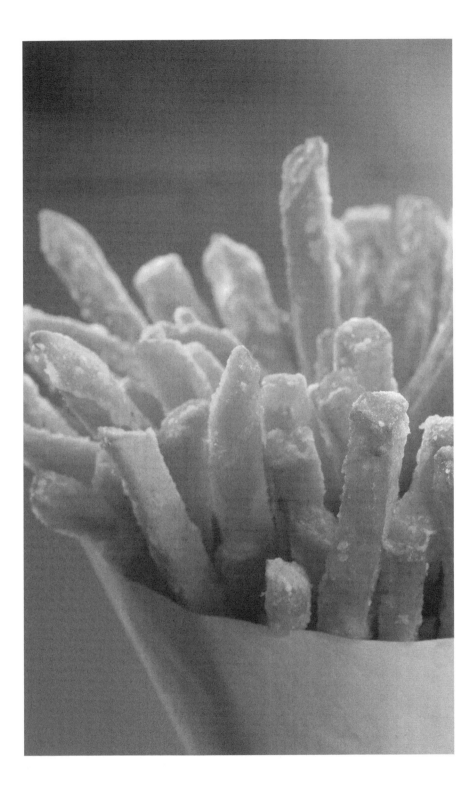

Paleo Fries with Herbs

Great with chicken drumsticks or thighs, nothing can beat these fries. The natural flavors from the herbs offer a mouthwatering combination, and the fries act as a great way to soak up any sauces on your plate from your chicken.

- 1½ teaspoons oregano, finely chopped
- 1½ teaspoons parsley, finely chopped
- ½ teaspoon thyme, finely chopped
- 4 large sweet potatoes, peeled and cut into evenly sized strips
- 1½ teaspoons ground pepper
- 2 tablespoons coconut oil, melted

Preheat oven to 425 degrees F. Place the oven rack in the middle position.

Combine all of the herbs, pepper, and sweet potatoes in a gallon-size freezer bag. Toss well to disperse the herbs evenly and then add the coconut oil.

Lay potatoes on a baking sheet in an even layer. Sprinkle the herb mixture on top.

Bake for 25 minutes, and then flip the potatoes around to cook for approximately another 15 to 20 minutes.

Serve hot.

Serves 4

Easy Garlic Butter Sauce

This sauce is easy to make and makes plain chicken breasts or vegetables perk up instantly. Store leftovers in the refrigerator and warm a little in the microwave if necessary.

- ¼ cup olive or coconut oil
- 2 cloves garlic, minced
- Freshly ground black pepper, to taste
- 1 tablespoon finely chopped fresh parsley

Heat a small saucepan over medium heat. Add the oil. Add the garlic and cook for about 2 minutes, until it starts to turn brown. Remove from heat.

Season with freshly ground black pepper. Stir in the parsley and serve.

Makes ¼ cup

Mango Chutney

This is a yummy dish that works well with grilled fish or chicken, and it goes wonderfully with crab cakes as well. Sweet and savory, you'll enjoy this with a variety of dishes. Make sure your mangoes are ripe before trying this recipe, otherwise you won't get the full flavor.

- 1 tablespoon coconut oil
- 1 garlic clove, minced
- 1 tablespoon fresh ginger, chopped
- ½ small red onion, minced
- 1 red bell pepper, chopped
- 2 ripe mangoes, pitted and chopped
- Juice of 1 lime
- 1 tablespoon curry powder
- 1 teaspoon red pepper flakes
- Freshly ground black pepper, to taste

In a small saucepan, heat the coconut oil over medium heat. Add the garlic and ginger and sauté for 2 minutes.

Add the onion and bell pepper and cook for 2 more minutes.

Add the rest of the ingredients and continue cooking until softened, about 5 more minutes.

Simmer about 10 minutes. Serve.

Makes 3 cups

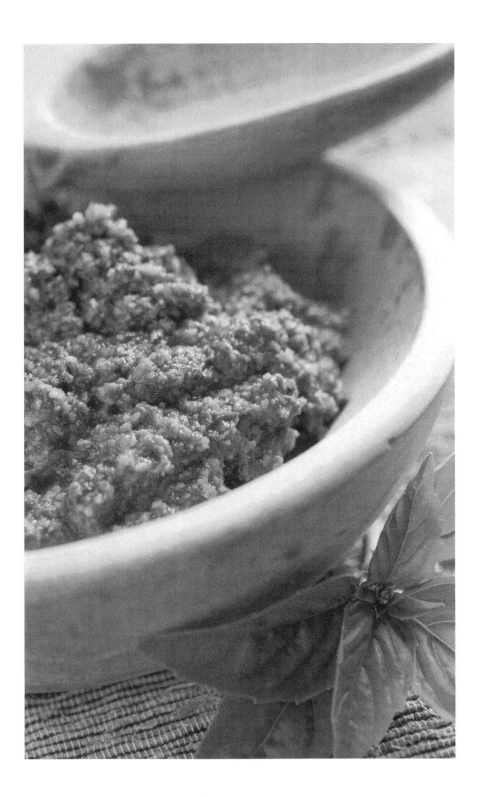

Paleo Pesto

Pesto is a popular Italian sauce that uses basil for the base. While it traditionally includes cheese, this version skips it. We don't think you'll miss it though. Try using other herbs for a variety of flavors. Mint and cilantro work especially well.

- 2 cups packed fresh basil leaves
- ½ cup walnuts
- ½ cup olive oil
- Juice of 1 lemon
- Freshly ground black pepper, to taste

Put the basil in a food processor and pulse until well chopped. Add the walnuts and continue chopping.

Slowly stream in the olive oil and lemon juice and puree until you have a smooth sauce. Season with freshly ground black pepper.

Refrigerate any leftover sauce.

Makes 2 cups

10

DESSERTS AND SNACKS

Paleo Chocolate Chip Cookies

What kind of dessert section would this be without chocolate chip cookies? Not a very good one, if we do say so ourselves. This recipe does not adhere to super strict Paleo standards, but it is grain free and does not contain any refined sugar. Because of this, they may not be as sweet as you might be used to, but we think that once you try them, you'll realize that it's sweet enough for a satisfying treat on a special occasion — just the way a dessert should be.

- 3 cups almond flour
- 1 teaspoon baking soda
- 2 large eggs
- ¼ cup pure maple syrup
- 1 teaspoon pure vanilla extract
- ½ cup coconut oil
- 1 cup bittersweet chocolate chips

Preheat oven to 375 degrees F.

Sift together the dry ingredients in a medium mixing bowl. Beat in the eggs, maple syrup, vanilla, and coconut oil with a hand mixer until well combined.

Fold in the chocolate chips.

On a parchment-lined baking sheet, drop tablespoon-sized balls of cookie dough about 2 inches apart. Bake for 15 minutes. Remove from oven, cool, and serve.

Makes 2 dozen

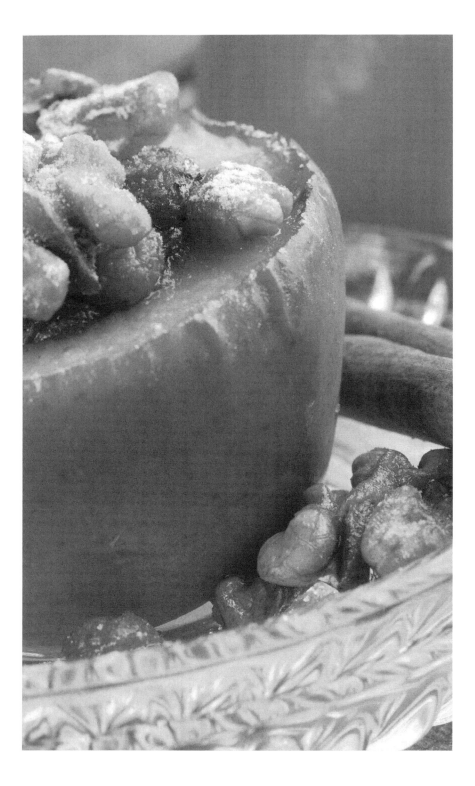

Baked Apples

You can treat these baked apples as either a dessert or a breakfast treat. You'll find the best cooking apples in mid to late fall. Choose tart but sweet varieties that have a firm texture. Try Winesap, Gravenstein, Jonagold, Fuji, or Pink Lady apples.

- 4 large baking apples
- Juice and zest of 1 lemon
- 3 tablespoons olive or coconut oil
- 3 tablespoons honey
- 1 teaspoon cinnamon
- ½ cup raisins
- ½ cup chopped walnuts

Preheat oven to 350 degrees F. Wash and core the apples.

Mix the remaining ingredients in a small bowl. Stuff the apples with the mixture.

Place the apples on a baking sheet and bake for 30 minutes, or until tender.

Serves 4

Raspberry Muffins

Raspberries add tart flavor and a chewy texture to these hearty muffins. Raspberries are in season in early summer, and again in fall. They are highly perishable, though, and should be refrigerated and stored within a day. Substitute frozen raspberries if you like, but don't thaw them before stirring them into the batter.

- 2 large eggs
- 3 ripe bananas, mashed
- ½ cup applesauce
- 1 teaspoon vanilla extract
- 1¼ cups almond meal
- 2 teaspoons baking powder
- ¼ teaspoon baking soda
- ¼ teaspoon cinnamon
- ¼ cup flaxseed flour
- 1 cup raspberries

Preheat oven to 350 degrees F. Spray a muffin pan with cooking spray.

Combine the eggs, banana, applesauce, and vanilla extract in a large mixing bowl. Add the dry ingredients and mix gently.

Fold in the raspberries gently. Pour ½ cup batter in each muffin cup. Bake 20 to 30 minutes, or until browned.

Serves 6

Berry Tart

When making a dish that relies extensively on the flavor of berries—as this one does—it is best to wait until you can get the freshest and ripest berries possible. Not only will they be sweet enough that you won't need to add any sugar, but their flavor will be fresh and pronounced. If you must use out-of-season berries, you can add a tablespoon or so of honey to the berry mixture.

Filling:

- 4 cups fresh mixed berries of your choice
- 1 cup water
- Juice of 1 lemon

Crust:

- 1½ cups almond flour
- ¼ teaspoon baking soda
- ½ teaspoon cinnamon
- ¼ teaspoon nutmeg
- ¼ cup coconut oil
- 1 teaspoon pure vanilla extract

Preheat oven to 350 degrees F.

Heat berries, water, and lemon juice in a medium saucepan. Simmer for 15 minutes, stirring and mashing berries periodically.

While fruit is simmering, combine all ingredients for the crust together in a large bowl. When you have a stiff dough, press into a pie pan and bake for 10 minutes. Remove from oven and allow to cool for 5 minutes.

Add the berry mixture to the crust and refrigerate for 1 hour before serving.

Serves 6

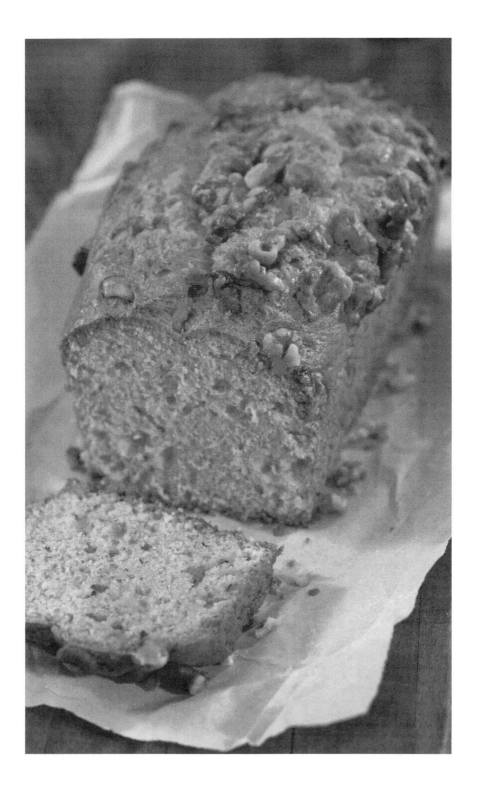

Banana Bread

Believe it or not, this loaf is baked without grains or wheat, and without sugar. Instead, the sweetness comes from very ripe bananas. When your banana skins are almost entirely black, that's when you know they'll be good in this recipe. While this is still not something you want to eat every single day, you can indulge in this tasty treat once in awhile without guilt.

- 3 cups almond flour
- 2 teaspoons baking soda
- 1 tablespoon cinnamon
- ¼ cup coconut oil
- 4 large eggs
- 2 large, very ripe bananas
- 1 tablespoon pure vanilla extract
- ½ cup walnuts, chopped and toasted

Preheat oven to 350 degrees F.

Sift the almond flour, baking soda, and cinnamon in a bowl. Add the rest of the ingredients and stir well to combine.

Pour the batter into a loaf pan greased with coconut oil. Bake for 25 to 28 minutes, until toothpick inserted in the center comes out clean.

Cool completely, remove from pan, and slice.

Serves 8 to 10

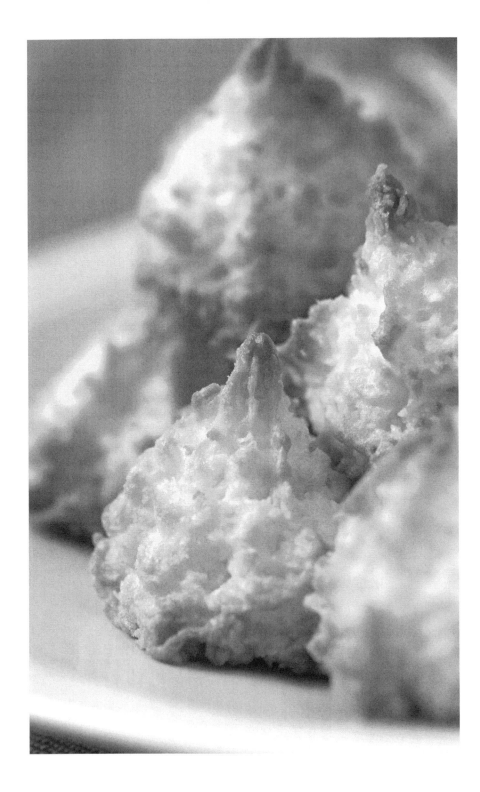

Coconut Macaroons

With only a few ingredients, these coconut treats are lightly sweet and surprisingly easy to whip up. Make sure to use unsweetened coconut so that you get the best flavor, and also no refined sugar. With hints of vanilla, these will bring a taste of the tropics to the end of your meal.

- 6 large egg whites
- ¼ cup pure maple syrup
- 1 teaspoon pure vanilla extract
- 3 cups shredded, unsweetened coconut

Preheat oven to 325 degrees F.

Beat the egg whites in a stand mixer until they form stiff peaks. Gently fold in the maple syrup, vanilla, and coconut.

Form into 1-inch balls and put on a parchment-lined baking sheet. Bake for 15 to 17 minutes, or until lightly browned.

Cool before serving.

Makes 1 dozen

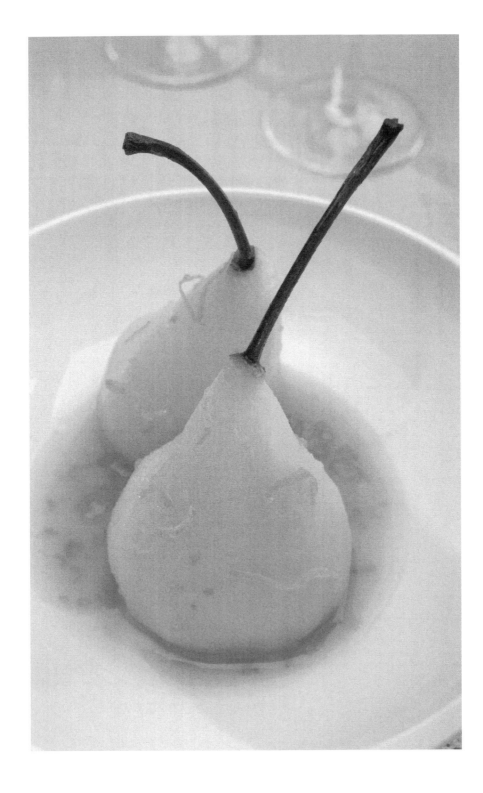

Poached Pears

Fruit makes a perfect dessert for the Paleo diet. It's sweet, but its natural sugar isn't bad for you the way that added sugars are. It's also high in fiber and nutrients, making it an even better choice. These poached pears make an elegant dessert for a dinner party and are easy to put together.

- Juice from 4 large oranges
- 1 small piece ginger, peeled
- 4 whole cloves
- 1 cinnamon stick
- 4 ripe but firm pears, such as Bosc, peeled and cored

Put all ingredients in a small saucepan and add enough water to ensure that the pears are just covered. If any parts of the pears are not covered in liquid, they will turn brown.

Bring to a boil and simmer on low for about 30 minutes. Remove pears.

Bring remaining liquid to a boil and reduce until it is thick and syrupy. Remove the cinnamon stick.

To serve, drizzle the warm pears with the syrup.

Serves 4

Primal Brownies

Like many of the dessert recipes you'll find here, these brownies are a better version of the classic dessert they're modeled after. They are more rich than sweet, and while they don't follow the Paleo principle strictly to the letter, they are close enough that we think they fit. As long as you don't eat the whole pan (it will be difficult!), you should be able to enjoy one of these every now and then without the guilt and remorse that comes with eating the real thing.

- 1 cup coconut oil
- 5 ounces bittersweet chocolate
- ½ cup pure maple syrup
- ¼ cup unsweetened cocoa powder
- 4 large eggs

- 1 teaspoon baking soda
- 1 tablespoon pure vanilla extract
- 1 cup raw, unsalted almond butter
- ¼ cup coconut flour

Preheat oven to 350 degrees F.

Mix the coconut oil, bittersweet chocolate, and maple syrup in a small saucepan over low heat. When melted and combined, remove from heat.

Add in the cocoa powder, stir, and set aside.

With a wooden spoon, blend in the eggs, baking soda, and vanilla. Add in the almond butter and stir until combined.

Fold in the coconut flour.

Pour batter into a 9 x 13-inch baking dish that has been lightly greased with coconut oil. Bake for 30 minutes.

Cool completely before cutting and serving.

Makes 1 dozen brownies

Caveman Trail Mix

Trail mix is full of antioxidants and protein for energy, making it a great on-the-go breakfast for the Paleo dieter. Substitute your favorite combination of nuts and dried fruit, and pack it in individual bags to grab quickly on busy mornings. Trail mix makes a great post-workout or sports practice food, too.

- 2 cups shredded coconut flakes
- ½ cup dried apricots, apples, blueberries, goji berries, or cherries, or a combination
- ½ cup chopped pecans, walnuts, or macadamia nuts
- ¼ cup cocoa

Combine all ingredients in a large mixing bowl. Store in an airtight container for up to one month.

Serves 4

Paleo Spiced Nuts

Nuts are a great snack when on the Paleo diet, but sometimes you want something more interesting than plain-old roasted nuts. These crunchy and toasty morsels fit the bill perfectly. Use any combination of nuts you like or have on hand—what's in the recipe is just a suggestion. Make sure that whatever you use is raw and unsalted.

- ½ cup whole almonds
- ½ cup walnuts
- ¼ cup sunflower seeds
- ¼ cup pumpkin seeds
- ¼ cup pecans, chopped
- ¼ cup pistachios

- 1 teaspoon dried rosemary
- 1 teaspoon dried thyme
- ¼ teaspoon cayenne pepper
- 1 tablespoon olive oil

Preheat oven to 350 degrees F.

Put everything in a gallon-size freezer bag. Shake to make sure all nuts are coated thoroughly with the oil and spices.

Lay on a parchment-lined baking sheet in an even layer and bake for 12 to 15 minutes, or until nuts are toasted. Cool completely before serving.

Makes 2 cups

Turkey Avocado Rollups

Finding healthy and easy snacks is difficult no matter what kind of diet you're on. While you have lots of options on the Paleo plan, sometimes you need something that is similar to a meal, but not huge. These rollups are almost like eating a turkey and avocado sandwich.

- 1 ripe avocado, peeled and pitted
- 1 tablespoon lemon juice
- 4 cherry tomatoes, roughly chopped
- Freshly ground black pepper, to taste
- 4 slices thick-cut turkey breast

Put the avocado and lemon juice in a bowl and mash thoroughly with a fork. Gently add in the tomatoes. Season with freshly ground black pepper.

Spread the avocado mixture on the turkey slices and roll up. Serve and enjoy!

Serves 1

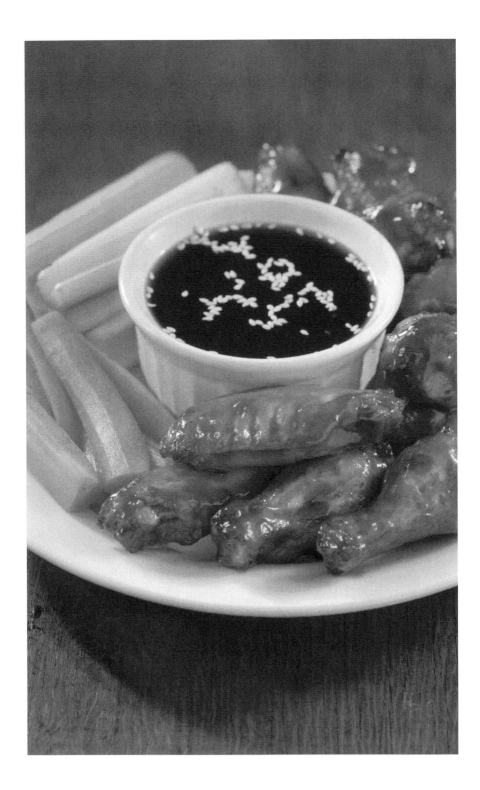

Teriyaki Chicken Drumsticks

Toss this simple dish in your slow cooker in the morning, and by dinner, you'll have tender, flavorful, Asian-inspired chicken that the whole family will love. Substitute whole, cut-up chicken for the drumsticks if you prefer.

- 8 chicken drumsticks
- ½ cup orange juice
- ½ cup coconut aminos
- ½ teaspoon ginger
- ½ teaspoon garlic
- Freshly ground black pepper, to taste

Place the drumsticks in the slow cooker and turn the slow cooker to low. Combine the remaining ingredients in a small bowl. Pour this mixture over the drumsticks. Cover and cook for 5 to 6 hours, or until tender. Turn occasionally so the chicken is thoroughly coated with the sauce.

Serves 4

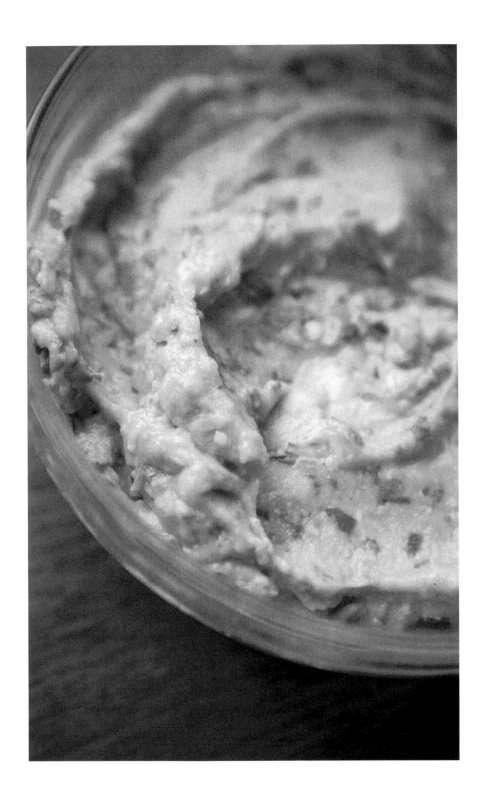

Fresh Guacamole

This easy, crowd-pleasing dip is one that is healthy as long as you don't eat it with a bunch of fried chips. Instead, try it with some veggies — peppers, celery, carrots, and cucumbers work well. If you're going to store it, squeeze some more lime juice over the top before putting in the refrigerator to keep it from browning.

- 2 ripe avocados, peeled and pitted
- 1 medium tomato, seeded and chopped
- ½ small red onion, diced
- 2 tablespoons fresh cilantro, chopped
- 1 clove garlic, minced
- Freshly ground black pepper, to taste
- Juice of 1 lime

In a medium bowl, mash the avocados with a fork until creamy, leaving as few chunks as possible.

Add in the tomatoes, onions, cilantro, and garlic. Season with freshly ground black pepper. Stir gently to combine and add the lime juice. Serve immediately.

Serves 6 to 8

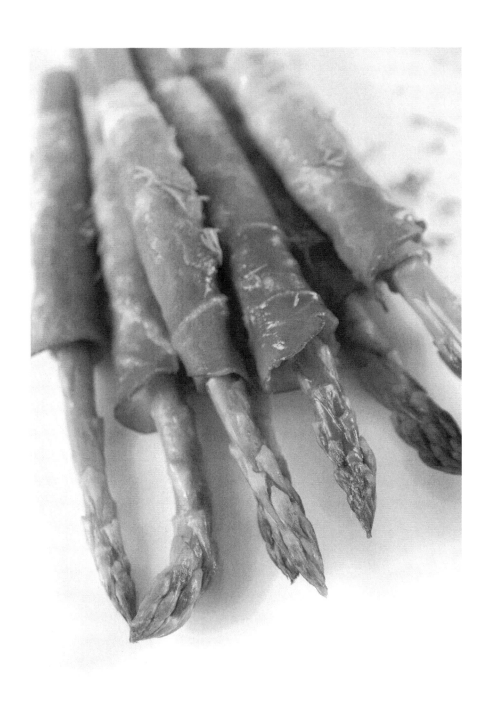

Prosciutto-Wrapped Asparagus

This is an easy appetizer that comes together fast. These work well for everything from casual gatherings to fancy dinner parties, and your guests are sure to love them. Get the highest quality prosciutto you can afford for the best flavor.

- 1 pound asparagus spears
- ¼ pound prosciutto, thinly sliced
- ½ medium onion, thinly sliced
- Freshly ground black pepper, to taste

Preheat oven to 400 degrees F. Slice the asparagus into 4-inch pieces.

Lay the prosciutto slices on a sheet pan and lay a few onion slices and asparagus pieces on each slice. Season with freshly ground black pepper. Roll them up, tucking the flap down.

Serves 8

Caveman Hummus

While hummus is traditionally made with chickpeas—a strict no-no on the Paleo diet—this version is made with zucchini. It's still creamy and delicious, and it's likely your guests won't know they aren't getting all those extra carbs.

- 2 medium zucchini
- ¾ cup tahini
- ¼ cup olive oil
- Juice of 2 lemons
- 2 garlic cloves, minced
- 1 tablespoon ground cumin
- Freshly ground black pepper, to taste
- Veggies, such as sliced bell peppers, tomatoes, carrots, and cucumbers, for serving

---

Peel and chop the zucchini and put in a food processor. Process until smooth.

Add the tahini, olive oil, lemon juice, garlic, and cumin and puree until creamy smooth. Season with freshly ground black pepper. Serve with sliced veggies for dipping.

Serves 6 to 8

CONCLUSION

Your decision to go on the Paleo diet has the potential to open a whole new world of vitality, health and delicious foods. Your continued determination to make changes to your lifestyle can ultimately lead to a longer, fuller and more active life.

If times get tough as you're following the Paleo diet, try to keep a positive attitude and remember that healthy habits can take time to become a seamless part of your daily life. Don't beat yourself up when you slip, and don't forget to reward yourself when you get back up. The potential for the Paleo diet to benefit your health, mind, energy levels and weight makes your commitment worthwhile.

Good luck on your journey back to your dietary roots!

INDEX